Print ALL the recipes

Want to get all the delicious recipes inside?

Don't want to hold your Kindle, iPad, iPhone, etc. while you are cooking in the kitchen?

Well **CLICK HERE** and get all the recipes contained inside this book in PDF and ready to PRINT.

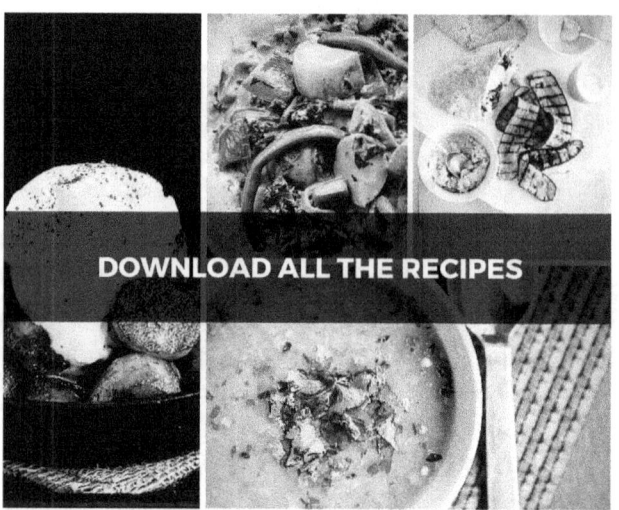

DOWNLOAD ALL THE RECIPES

Introduction

"Why would you do that to yourself?!"

That's the first thing my friends and family said to me when I told them I wanted to go vegan.

For most people not familiar with animal cruelty, the climate impact of animal agriculture and the adverse health effects of SAD (Standard American Diet), we can often seem like crazy people.

Of course, if you are reading this you know that this is not the case. I myself have been able to put away my enjoyment of eating animals in the name of protecting them and the environment.

Along the way, I've established a love for vegan foods and my palette has slowly changed to adapt to this new way of eating.

So here is my story about how I came upon this diet, why I've chosen it for myself, the challenges I faced along the way and finally why I've come to write this book.

———

Click here to download all recipes and other bonuses

Brainwashed to Change

In August 2014, I was your typical meat eater. I needed to have one piece of meat with each meal - whether it was chicken, fish or a big steak.

One day, I happened to come across Fork Over Knives on Netflix and sat down to watch it with my girlfriend one night and after that movie my perspective on eating meat dramatically shifted.

I love to consume information so I quickly went about devouring a dozen of other documentaries on the same subject (which you should checkout yourself) - movies like:

• Vegucated (NetFlix)

• Earthlings (YouTube)

• Fat, Sick & Nearly Dead (Part 1 + 2)

• Hungry for Change (NetFlix)

• Food Matters (NetFlix)

• Cowspiracy (Netflix)

• King Corn (NetFlix)

• Fed Up (NetFlix)

Yes - I really went in headfirst but I think it is necessary because our entire culture revolves around the consumption of animals and their byproducts.

We are told since we are infants that you need to drink your milk and are fed delicious ice cream and extravagant meals built on top of the death and destruction of animals.

It was necessary to reverse that programming and going deep into the world of veganism with these documentaries allowed me to see all the destruction I was causing with my choices.

So one day after watching a few too many, I called up my girlfriend and told her I wanted to switch - she told me she would join me and we got started on September 1st.

The Fake Meat Era

To start out with I didn't want to put the effort in to make my own meals, so we often found ourselves eating out everyday at vegan restaurants.

We would find dishes with meat alternatives and just get our meat fix from these items.

Most people start out this way with meat alternatives like Soy, Seitan and Tofu among others which are just a poor mans version of meat.

While it may be better for the environment than eating meat, these highly processed foods are only meant to be side items and not the focal point of a vegan meal.

Eating too much you'll quickly find leads to a degeneration in your health.

So yes, you CAN be an unhealthy vegan BUT I also feel this is a natural progression for most meat eaters to a vegan diet.

So don't be alarmed if this is how you approach changing over. Your taste buds need time to adjust to this new palette.

Vegan Nirvana

My final stage is where I've learnt to be a largely whole food eater while limiting my intake of processed fake meats to side items on my dinner plate.

I've added a host of seeds and pseudo-grains to my diet which have put the necessary protein and amino acids that we require as vegans.

This change came after reading Brendan Brazier's "Thrive Diet" and even though it was very informative, there was something missing.

More specifically, the recipes inside were very complicated and the most basic questions about the diet were not answered.

Like what to buy and when, what fruits and vegetables can be kept outside the fridge, and what are the different types of seeds and why do we need each one.

Basically, I needed to know as a former meat eater the most basic things about a vegan diet.

That's where this book comes in.

Inside, we've put together simple recipes that can be made in minutes NOT hours so when you get that craving you can quickly slap something together.

We've looked at the most common mistakes new vegans make and what happens when you don't get enough calories for instance.

Here's a quick rundown of what you'll find:

- The 15 key ingredients EVERY vegan should keep around their house

- The 5 biggest mistakes NEW vegans almost always make when they start

- What fruits, vegetables, seeds and grains can be refrigerated / left out / put in the freezer and how long they each will last

- 15 sublime tips to wow your friends when hosting your FIRST ever vegan dinner party

- How to ripen a banana in ONLY 20 minutes

This book is everything I wish I had known when I first started on this journey.

So here's to a healthier, easier transition to a new diet that will change your life.

Imran

Fantastic Tofu Scramble

Tofu, also known as bean curd, is an ingredient every vegan needs to always have in the kitchen.

I often have several packets in my fridge (or the freezer) which I can quickly cut up, cook and toss onto salads, into soups and put into almost every dish imaginable.

Tofu is not only cruelty-free, but also a great source of protein and all the eight essential amino acids.

For a good start, here is a basic tofu scramble recipe you can make in only 15 minutes.

This recipe makes two servings, with each serving less than 400 Calories.

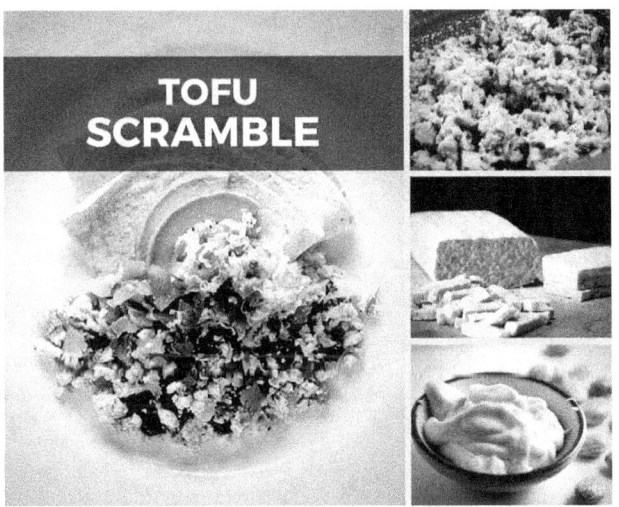

Ingredients

- 1/2 onion, diced

- 1/2 green bell pepper, diced

- 1 block tofu, drained and pressed

- 2 tbsp coconut oil or margarine

- 1 tsp onion powder

- 1 tsp garlic powder

- 1 tbsp soy sauce

- 2 tbsp nutritional yeast

- 1/2 tsp turmeric (op-tional)

Preparation

First, ready your tofu for the draining and pressing process.

Like in most tofu dishes, the best-tasting tofu is achieved when it is drained and pressed.

When you skip this process, the tofu will fail to absorb the flavours and the seasonings you add it.

Don't know how to press tofu? Read on.

Pressing Tofu

- Paper towels

- Cutting board

- Heavy objects

1. Fold a paper towel in half or quarters. Place it

in the middle of the cutting board.

2. Put the tofu on the folded paper towel. Make sure that the paper towels can absorb a large amount of moisture.

3. Fold another paper towel and put it on top of the tofu.

4. Place heavy objects on the tofu and leave it for 15 to 30 minutes.

Preparation

After pressing, slice the tofu into cubes then crumb it to your desired consistency using a fork or your hand.

Then, heat a large pan and sauté the chopped onion, crumbled tofu and green bell pepper in coconut oil or margarine for about 5 minutes.

Stir frequently.

Next, turn the heat down then add the soy sauce, garlic powder and onion powder.

Let it cook for five more minutes, stirring frequently. You can add a little oil if you like.

Lastly, add the nutritional yeast. Stir well to make sure that your tofu is well coated with the yeast.

Make it AWESOME

You can eat the tofu scramble as it is. But if you want a better tofu scramble experience, you can serve it wrapped in tortilla for a breakfast burrito.

You can also add vegan meat, mushrooms and spinach the next time you make one.

With tofu, there are so many ingredients that you can mix and match and still keep it delicious (and healthy) in the end.

--

Want to print this recipe? <u>Click here</u>

More Simple Recipes…

If you are interested in super simple recipes (like the one above) but with only 8 ingredients in each recipe, then you have to check out <u>thevegan8.com</u>.

Brandi, the founder of <u>Vegan8</u>, has done a fantastic job of creating delicious recipes that will simplify your shopping trip.

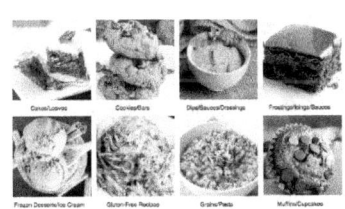 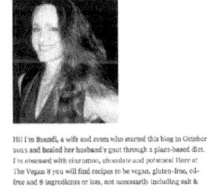

There's even a sections for kids and for people with allergies!

15 Key Ingredients Vegans Should Keep in the House

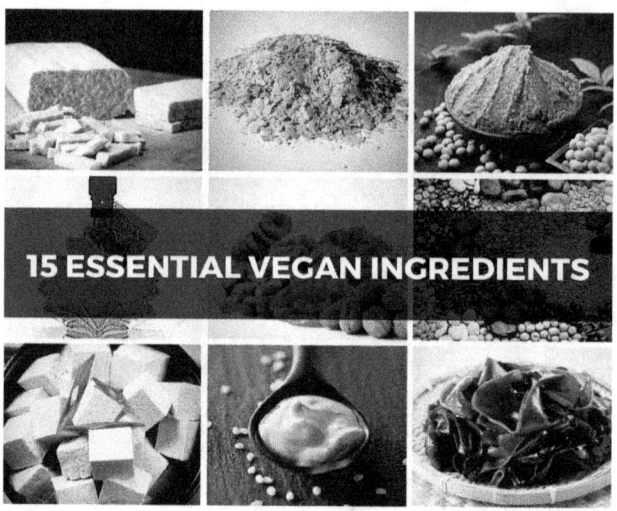

One of the biggest challenges I had going vegan was figuring out what to buy and keep around the house.

There are so many options from Tofurky to Kidney Beans to Arame Seaweed - you can quickly end up going broke stocking your shelves with everything.

To get you over the intimidation factor, this list will give you the **15 essential ingredients I keep around the house.**

Although vegans have different preferences in taste, ethnic backgrounds, and of course, allergies, these ingredients are all helpful in adding protein, flavour, colour and texture to your everyday food.

1. Beans

    It's great to have a variety of beans at home as they are nice add-ons to soups, salads and stews, pasta dishes and even

pilafs. Lentils and chickpeas make good addi-
tions to almost any dish.
Other beans I common-
ly buy are black, mung,
pinto, kidney, anasai and
cannellini beans.

2.   Grains

Grains provide nutri-
tional boost, a good
amount of iron, flavour
and texture to vegan
meals. Make sure to al-
ways have brown rice,
oat groats, quinoa, mil-

let, spelt, barley and bul-

gur.

3. Tofu

For non-vegans, tofu is
regarded as a boring,
tasteless food. But for
vegans, it is an essential,
protein-rich part of
their diet. It may be
tasteless but it works
by absorbing flavour
and texture to everyday
vegan food. It can be
used in many different
dishes, and can even be
used in desserts.

4. Tempeh

    Read as "tehm-pay," it is just like tofu but fermented. To make tempeh, fry or grill the tempeh with a variety of seasonings to be savoury. Aside from tofu, it is one of the best sources of protein for us vegans. *When stored in a freezer, it can last for a couple of months.*

5. Miso

    A Japanese paste from fermented soya, miso

can improve the taste of a wide range of dishes. Miso paste vary in colour, corresponding to different levels of savouriness. It is commonly used in soups and as salad dressing.

6. Tahini

Tahini is a bitter paste made from ground sesame. It is very rich in calcium and goes well with miso. Together, they can make tofu, tempeh and steamed vegetables a lot more interesting.

7.   Nuts

Aside from protein, nuts are valuable sources of calcium and magnesium. You can throw them into salads, pastas and stir-fries to add a little flavour and life to the dish. *Almonds, walnuts, cashews, hazelnuts and pecans' shelf life can be extended by storing them in the freezer.*

8. Dried fruits

Many think dried fruits
are only for snack time.
What they don't realize
is that dried fruits like
apricots, figs, berries
and raisins add a deli-
cious kick of flavour to
many dishes. They are
now a staple to give life
to my boring salads.

9. Vegetable stock

You can always make
your own vegetable
stock, but if you want

the easy road, just grab a few boxes at the supermarket.

10. Nutritional yeast

Nutritional yeast is used to create a cheesy consistency. It comes in flake or powdered form. It is usually added to soup or popcorn, or even used as *a cheese dip substitute just by mixing it with water.*

11. Seaweeds

Seaweeds are rich sources of many different vitamins and minerals. There are several kinds of seaweeds to choose from but most of the time they are used in Japanese recipes. Among them are nori, kombu and hijiki that enhance rice, soups and salads, respectively.

12. Flax seeds

Flax seeds are loaded with Omega-3 fatty acids, lignans and fiber that help reduce the risk of heart disease, stroke, cancer and diabetes. You can put them in your muffins, oats and even smoothies. Also, ground flax seed, when mixed with water, can be an egg substitute.

13. Coconut oil

This oil is known as one of the most versatile as it can be used in many dishes. It is also a great substitute for butter. Most importantly, it can last on the shelf for a very long time.

14. Spices and flavourings

Sea salt, black pepper and soy sauce are just some of the flavourings you need to always have in your vegan kitchen.

15. Maple syrup

Maple syrup is a favourite for me. It can be added to everything from breads to roasted squash and even sweet potato soup. And of course, who can forget pancakes? Other natural sweeteners are agave nectar and brown rice syrup.

It's Betta than Tuna Tempeh Salad

Want something done fast for lunch?

In just ten minutes, you will be able to taste this super yummy but healthy salad that makes four servings.

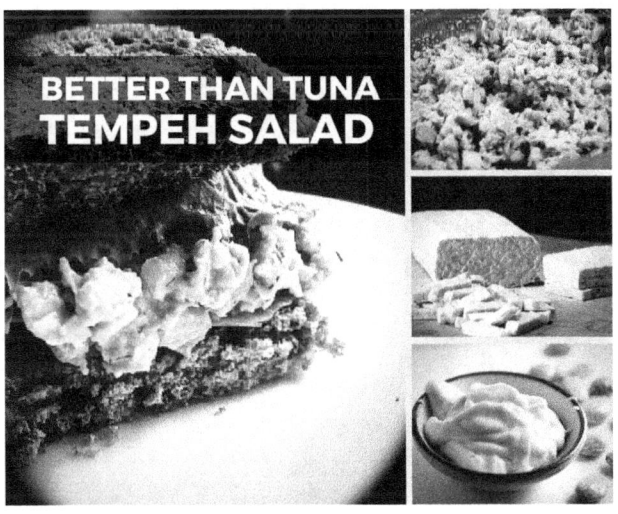

Ingredients

- 8 ounces tempeh, crum-bled

- ½ cup scallion (or red onion), finely chopped

- ½ cup celery, finely chopped

- ½ cup vegan mayonnai-se

- ½ teaspoon dried dill

- ½ teaspoon celery salt

- fresh black pepper

Preparation

1. Crumb your tempeh into small pieces.

2. Mix all ingredients in a bowl until they are evenly distributed.

3. Add celery salt and black pepper to taste.

4. Refrigerate until ready to serve.

5. You can serve it between whole wheat bread.

--

Want to print this recipe? <u>Click here</u>

Tempeh vs. Tofu vs. Soy: Busting Some Myths

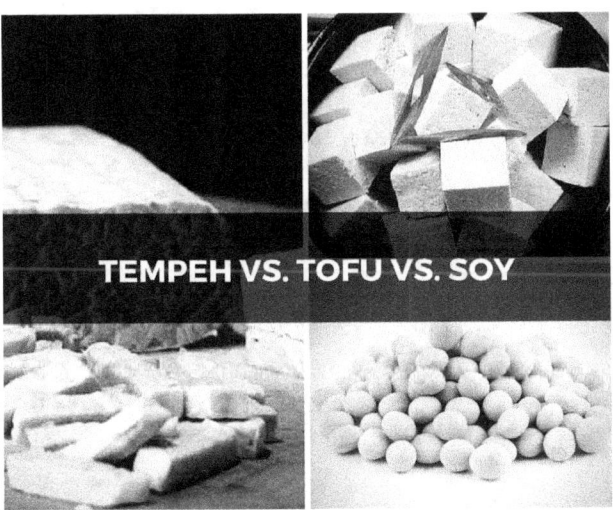

In the absence of meat in the vegan diet, vegans are always looking for new and delicious sources of protein.

Tofu and tempeh, both derived from soy, are now becoming household staples.

But what are tofu, tempeh and soy?

And among the things we hear about them, which ones are true?

Tofu and tempeh are close relatives from the soybean. Where they differ greatly is in their preparation.

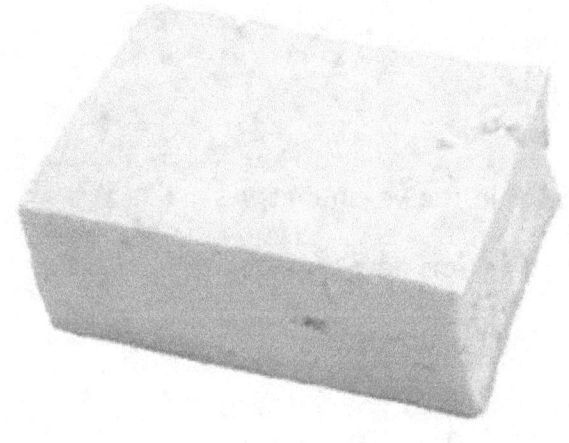

Tofu

Tofu is made from the pulp or curd of soy-beans after the soy milk has been made.

The pulp is then mixed with a coagulant or thickening agent in order to be made into chunks, bricks or slabs.

The process follows the same principle as when dairy milk is made into cottage cheese. A rich source of calcium, magnesium and iron, tofu is a great addition to your diet, vegan or not.

Tofu is also cholesterol-free, low in calories and contains little fat.

Tempeh

Tempeh, on the other hand, is a whole soybean product made from fermented soybeans. The soybeans are soaked until tender and then partially cooked.

After cooking, the soybean is made into a cake or patty form. Although there are other variations of tempeh available in the market, soy tempeh is still the most common variety.

Tempeh has a hearty texture and is a complete protein. **In fact, it has more than double the protein content of tofu.**

A 100-gram serving of tempeh has *19 grams of protein while the same amount of tofu has only 8 grams of protein.*

Therefore, tempeh is better for you if you need a protein boost.

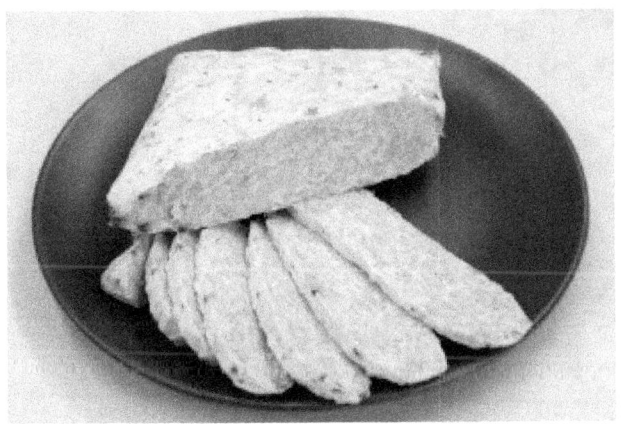

The fermentation process that tempeh undergoes preserves the whole bean, increasing its protein, fibre and vitamin content.

Tofu and tempeh may sound very promising for your health, but there are a lot of allegations about the harms they, specifically soy products, may cause.

Here are some of them:

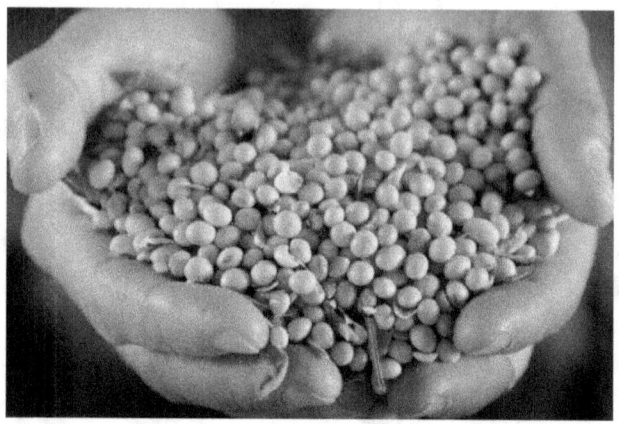

Myth: All soy is genetically modified organisms (GMOs).

Fact: While it is true that a large percentage of soybean crops are GMOs (81 percent) and 85 percent of that is fed to farmed animals, there are still organic soybean products available in the market today.

Myth: Soy consumption causes man boobs.

Fact: Let's face it - a lot of people think this.

However, studies show that frequent soy consumption will not affect your testosterone level or lead to Gynecomastia (man boobs technical term) in men.

The confusion comes from people thinking phytoestrogen, which is found in soy (and all meat, dairy, eggs for that matter), is the same as estrogen.

It is not. And it has completely different effects on the body.

It's all rather complicated but you can read more here

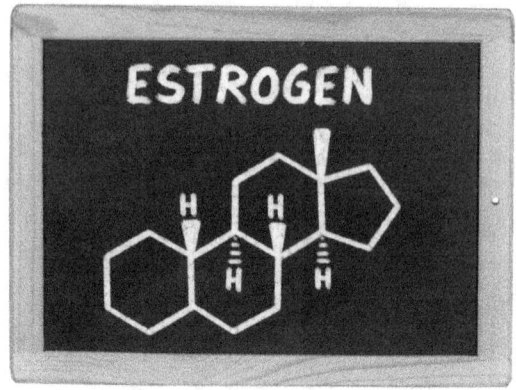

Myth: Soy causes cancer.

Fact: As mentioned, Phytoestrogen is different from Estrogen. Estrogen is a natural hormone that proliferates cell growth which can lead to a higher risk of cancer.

On the other hand, Phytoestrogen is weakly Estrogenic or Antiestrogenic. Isoflavones, a Phytoestrogen, in soy do not have the Estrogenic effect of inducing tumour growth.

In fact, Isoflavones protect the body against hormone-dependent types of cancer.

Whew…heavy stuff, now time for another recipe.

Raw Tabouli Hemp Seed Salad

Now that you already know the nutritional value of soy, tofu and tempeh, I will now introduce you to a seed that can power up day.

This recipe's key ingredient is the hemp seed -- a superfood containing a large amount of plant protein and Omega 3 fatty acids.

Just three tablespoons of this seed, will get you an *astounding 11 grams of protein.*

Hemps seeds not only make you healthy inside, but also makes you beautiful outside as an effect of the minerals magnesium, zinc, iron and phosphorus they contain.

This salad also has parsley, an herb that is packed with iron and Vitamins A and C. It is a digestive aid, natural diuretic and blood purifier which prevents diseases.

You can make this refreshing salad, which serves 2, in 15 minutes or less.

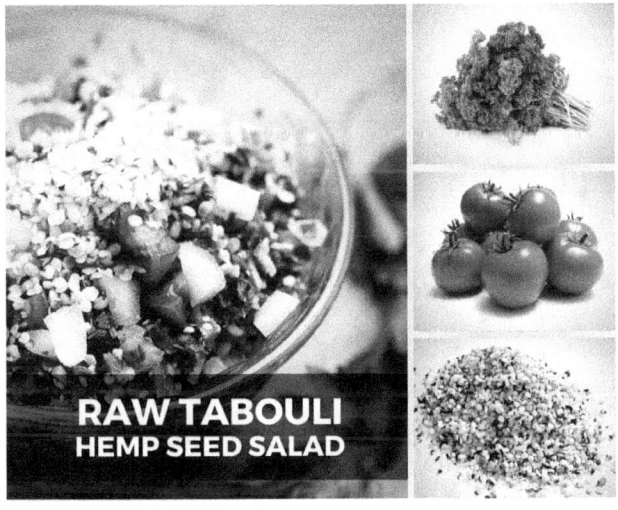

RAW TABOULI
HEMP SEED SALAD

Ingredients

Base:

- 1 huge bunch of parsley (curly or Italian flat)

- 1 organic tomato, diced

- 6 heaping tbs. of hemp seeds

- ½ white onion, diced

Dressing:

- Juice of 1 lemon

- 1 clove of garlic, minced

- Cold-pressed olive oil

- Sea salt, to taste

Preparation

1. Chop the parsley and throw it into a large bowl.

2. Add the onion, tomato and hemp seeds.

3. Combine the lemon, olive oil, garlic and sea salt.

4. Blend or mix well.

5. Pour over the salad and mix well.

--

Want to print this recipe? Click here

BONUS TIME: Another minimalist kitchen…

Amanda and Aaron run Picklesnhoney.com out of Boston, MA and it's another great vegan blog.

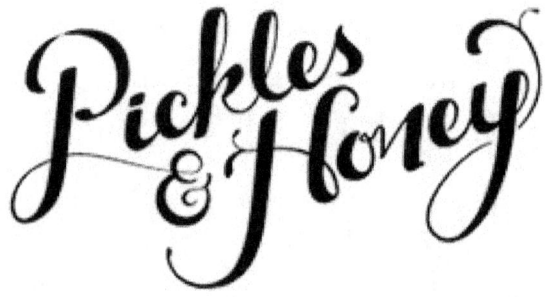

In the theme of this book, they are minimalist chefs focusing on recipes with 10 or less ingredients.

Definitely check them out if you want to add to your minimalist recipe collection.

The Showdown of the Seeds

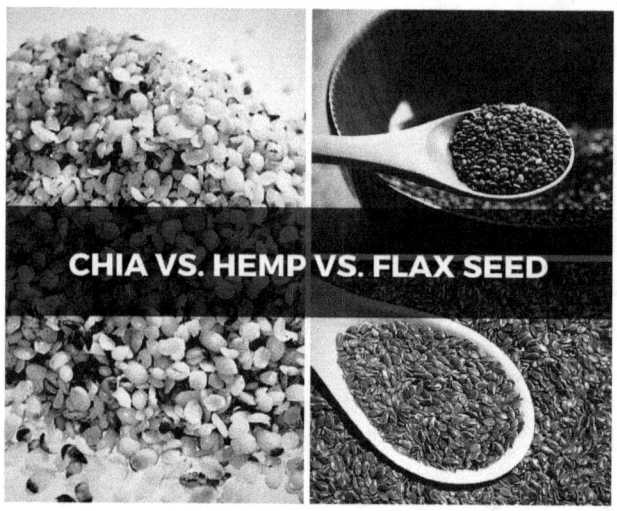

CHIA VS. HEMP VS. FLAX SEED

You already know that there are superfood seeds you can add to your pantry for more health benefits and one of them is the hemp seed.

There are two other tiny superfoods: the chia seed and the flax seed and you will know about them as you read through.

You will also learn more about the hemp seed and what are the similarities and differences between the 3.

Chia Seeds

Chia is a member of the mint family that is native to Guatemala and Mexico.

Although chia seeds seem to be gaining popularity around the world just recently, they have been known as very important food crops by the Aztecs during their time.

The white and dark brown/black varieties are the ones recommended for consumption.

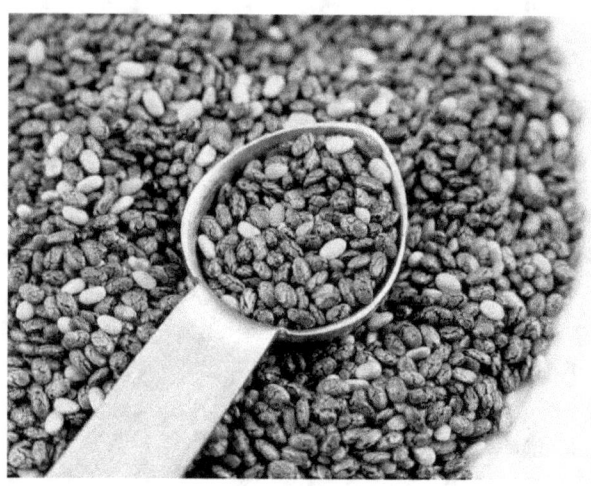

Chia seeds may be tiny, but the health effects and benefits they offer are very significant.

An ounce (28 grams) of these seeds has 11 grams of dietary fibre which will keep your digestive health in the best shape.

They are also a great source of Omega 3 fatty acids important for brain health.

In fact, chia's Omega 3 conversion into the body beats flax seeds'.

These seeds also make a great source of protein, with 4.4 grams per ounce of serving. They also have calcium, manganese, and phosphorus for stronger teeth and bones.

Chia is also proven to eliminate belly fat due to insulin resistance.

Other positive health effects include boosting energy, stabilizing blood sugar, lowering cholesterol, and improving heart health.

Chia seeds are generally tasteless, so they won't affect your foods' flavour.

That means you can add it to whatever food you are eating, even ice cream! Some people also feed their pets chia seeds, making their coats shiny and lush.

The seeds can be eaten whole or milled.

However, Wayne Coates, the researcher who is responsible for bringing fame to chia seeds in North America, suggests avoiding red and smaller than regular black chia seeds as they are not safe for consumption.

Hemp Seeds

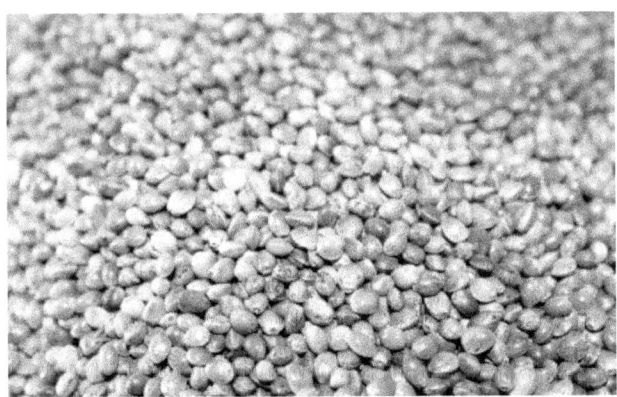

Hemp seeds come from the hemp plant, Cannabis sativa L. Contrary to popular belief, hemp seeds are different from marijuana.

I should point out that **hemp seeds will not make you high** as it contains less than 1 percent delta-9-tetrahydrocannabinol or THC.

Marijuana contains 20 percent.

Major producers are Canada, France and China but it has been banned in the US since the 1950s.

Hemp seeds can be sterilized, roasted, toasted, or cracked. They can be pressed into oil or hulled into meal. They have an amazing nutty flavour that can easily blend with any dish.

Oil extracted from seeds can also be incorporated into any meal, or even taken as is.

Hemp seeds are said to have the most concentrated balance of proteins, vitamins, essential fats, and enzymes combined with a relative absence of sugar, starches and satu-

rated fats.

In fact, they contain 20 different varieties of

amino acids and all nine essential amino

acids our bodies cannot produce.

Four tablespoons (42 grams) of hemp seeds

contain the following:

- 15 g protein

- 2.5 g fiber

- 4.5 g carbohydrates

- No cholesterol

They can also control blood sugar, reduce

the risk of getting colon and prostate cancer, treat tuberculosis and aid in the healing process of diseases.

They have a perfect 3:1 ratio of Omega-6 Linoleic Acid and Omega-3 Linolenic Acid – for cardiovascular health and general strengthening of the immune system.

Hemps seeds thrive almost anywhere, under a variety of environmental conditions, and are rarely affected by pests or disease.

They are considered to be allergy-free and are safe to be consumed by pets.

Keep the seeds cool when in storage.

When preparing food, add the seeds after cooking as heat destroys the nutritional effects of the fatty acids.

Flax Seed

Flax seeds have been around for centuries and today, they can be found in all kinds of food.

If your egg has a higher level of Omega 3 fatty acids, then the chicken who laid it must be fed with flax seeds.

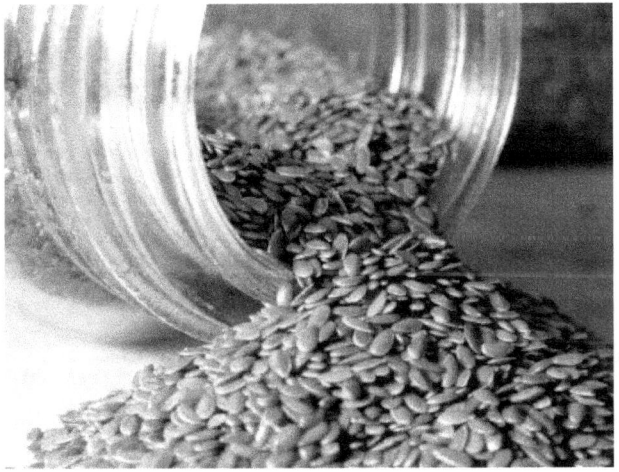

Doctors suggest to ground the flax seeds before eating to be able to easily absorb the health benefits.

Flaxseed has three primary components namely Omega-3, fiber and lignan.

What do these components do?

Like chia and hemp seeds, flax seeds also contain Omega-3 fatty acids also know as good fats.

Its main function is to protect and maintain the heart's health. Each tablespoon of flaxseed contains around 1.8 grams of Omega-3.

On the other hand, lignans have both estrogen and antioxidant qualities. Lignan content in flaxseed is 75 to 800 times more than other plant foods.

Lignans are also found to protect against tumour growth by blocking enzymes associated with it.

Same with the other two seeds, flax seeds help fight heart disease, lung disease diabetes and breast, colon and prostate cancer.

They also lower blood pressure and reduce inflammation.

In animal studies, the plant omega-3 fatty acid found in flaxseed, called ALA, inhibited tumour incidence and growth.

The Flax Council of Canada suggests 1 to 2 tablespoons of ground flaxseed a day as the normal dosage.

However, pregnant and breastfeeding women should not supplement their diets with ground flax seeds until proven safe.

The brown flaxseed is the most common variety available in most supermarkets.

There is also a golden-coloured variety but there is very little difference in nutritional content between the two.

Keep whole flaxseed in a cool, dark place until you grind it.

But as long as it's dry, room temperature can do. For ground flaxseed, put them in a plastic bag and store them in the freezer.

To read more and to find all the sources for this information check out the following links:

- <u>The Benefits of Flaxseed</u>

- <u>Pure Healing Foods: Hemp Seeds</u>

- <u>Chia Seed Benefits: 10 Reasons to Add Chia to Your Diet</u>

Spicy Zucchini Pita Pockets

Got ten minutes?

Then you can quickly throw together this delicious meal that I probably have once per week.

Some nutritional facts for you; each serving gives you 21 grams of protein and 12 grams of fibre.

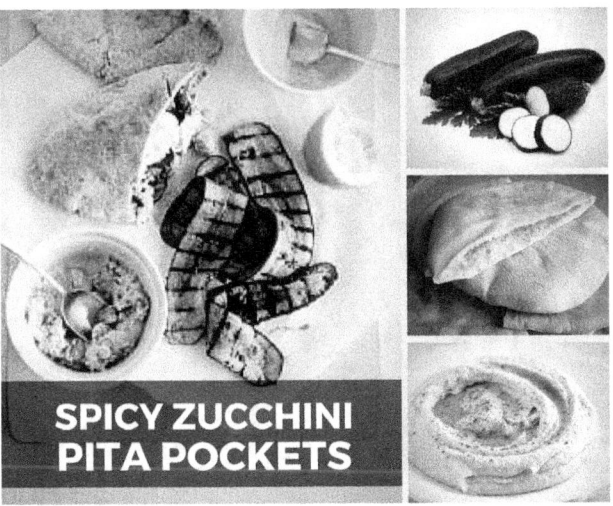

SPICY ZUCCHINI PITA POCKETS

Ingredients

- I zucchini, peeled and thinly sliced lengthwise

- broad beans

- I large pita bread

- I clove small garlic, crushed

- I spring onion, thinly sliced

- 2 Tbsp hummus

- 2 tsp harissa paste

- I tsp tahini paste

- I tbsp vegan yogurt

- Juice of I lemon

- 2 tsp coconut oil

- Preparation

Preparation

On a hot pan with coconut oil and Harissa, cook each side of the zucchini slices for 2 minutes. Once tender, transfer to a plate and set aside.

In a pot, heat water and wait until it boils. Add the broad beans and let it cook for 2 minutes. Once done, drain them under cold running water and remove their skins.

Mix the broad beans, spring onions and hummus in a small bowl. In another bowl, mix the tahini, lemon juice, garlic and Greek-style yogurt.

Toast the pita and split it to create two pockets. In each pocket, spread some hummus mix, put in the zucchini slice, then drizzle a little yogurt mixture.

Serve and enjoy!

--

Want to print this recipe? <u>Click here</u>

BONUS: Another Website with Easy to Make Items

Although not strictly a vegan website, the-boredvegetarian.com has a ton of awesome recipes.

Bethany Pickard makes my mouth water with her stunning images of the food she makes.

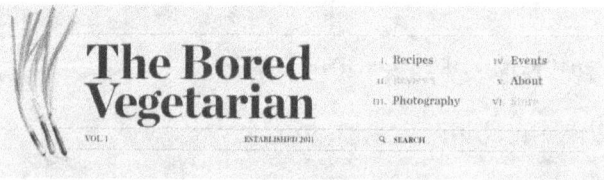

If you want a beautiful journey through a plant-based diet then check The Bored Vegetarian out.

Where to Find Vegan Products: 5 Top Spots On-line

The vegan lifestyle is clearly unfamiliar territory for those who came from a predominantly meat-based diet.

I think one of the biggest worries new vegans have when looking up new recipes is…

"Where do I get all this stuff?"

Good news, awareness on veganism is continuously growing and expanding, providing easier and faster access to many different vegan products.

As a result, more and more vegan shopping portals are coming online.

These websites serve as a marketplace for a wide range of products, from food items to household products and even cosmetics.

They provide a convenient way of searching and buying stuff that will satisfy your vegan needs — all in the comfort of your home.

Here are the my top 5:

Vegan Perfection

Vegan Perfection offers a variety of food items, vegan chocolate, candies and hemp oil-based body care products.

You can also find DVDs and books up for grabs, many of which you don't see every-day. What's great about the website is that it's easy to navigate.

Once you enter, you can quickly see what it offers, both from big labels and independent businesses.

Not only that, most of the vegan products are certified organic!

Now that's true perfection!

Shop Vegan

Shop Vegan distinguishes itself from others on this list by having more lifestyle products than items for your pantry.

If you're looking for supplements, body care, perfumes, condoms (yes! vegan), confectionery, and clothing, then you're in the right place.

They also post special offers and discounts for your favourite vegan products.

Shop Vegan is great for cosmetics and gift ideas, even for your furry friends.

Vegan Essentials

Being one of the biggest online shopping platforms for all things vegan, Vegan Essentials can provide almost all of your vegan needs.

Whether it's food, body care, fashion, supplements or pet products, it's all here.

———

Want 10% off

Use "veganorbust" during checkout - available until Jan 1st, 2016 on all products except cold shippers

Pangea The Vegan Store

An advocate of all cruelty-free products (humans + animals alike), Pangea The Vegan Store only offers goods that are manufactured in countries where workers are protected by labor laws and unions.

It has a very comprehensive range of products compared to some stores on this list.

From the usual food items, cosmetics and gift sets, it also sells home, office and cleaning products.

The website has a fresh, clean and positive vibe that will make your shopping experience a breeze.

Vegan Cuts

Vegan Cuts is a fantastic shopping destination largely focused around products for women.

The layout is cute, fun and fresh but at the same time offers a variety of vegan products with many different brands.

What sets it apart from others is that when you sign up, it will send a special deal to your email every week.

They also have a beauty box containing 4 to 7 different products you can subscribe to.

Go to Vegan Cuts if you're looking for food items, body care, clothing, shoes, and accessories.

Quick Veggie Curry

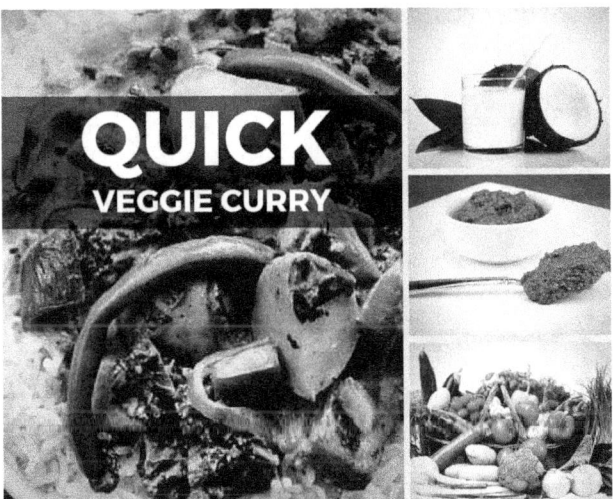

Ingredients

- 1-3 cups chopped fresh vegetables any kind you like

- 1 handful of spinach/ kale/chard, chopped

- 1 onion, thinly sliced

- 2 cloves garlic, crushed

- 1 tbsp fresh ginger, grated

- 2-3 tsp curry paste

- canola or olive oil

- 1 14 oz (398 mL) can
coconut milk

- chutney (optional)

- salt and pepper

- cumin

Preparation

Heat oil in a large skillet over medium-high heat. Sauté the onions until soft then add the garlic and ginger. Let it cook for a minute.

Next, add firm vegetables like cauliflower and potatoes, and cook until edges turn golden brown.

Then, put in the rest of the vegetables along with curry paste, salt, cumin and coconut milk. Mix well and wait until it simmers.

Pour in the chutney if you like and stir. Cook until the sauce thickens and the veg-etables tender.

Sprinkle some salt and pepper.

Lastly, add the spinach/kale/chard and cook until it wilts.

Serve over steamed rice.

--

Want to print this recipe? Click here

BONUS TIME: More Spicy Recipes

Being an indian, I absolutely love this blog full of amazing indian inspired vegan recipes.

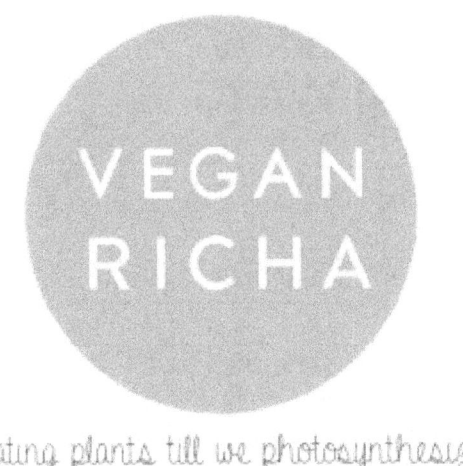

eating plants till we photosynthesize!

Richa Hingle has done a fantastic job giving you all your favourite indian recipes in vegan form without giving up on taste.

5 Biggest Mistakes New Vegans Almost ALWAYS Make

Just starting out in the vegan lifestyle?

At first, it will feel scary and daunting, just like how going to a place you know nothing about.

For myself, it was a monumental shift from a meat diet and there was not much guidance for complete newbies.

I ended up losing a ton of muscle mass and feeling tired and lethargic about 3 months in...if I hadn't been so passionate about the cause, I could have easily given up.

So, whether it is for health or ethical reasons that pushed you to make the switch, you have to be familiar with the biggest mistakes newbies make in order to avoid them.

Here are the five biggest mistakes new vegans make and tips on how to avoid them:

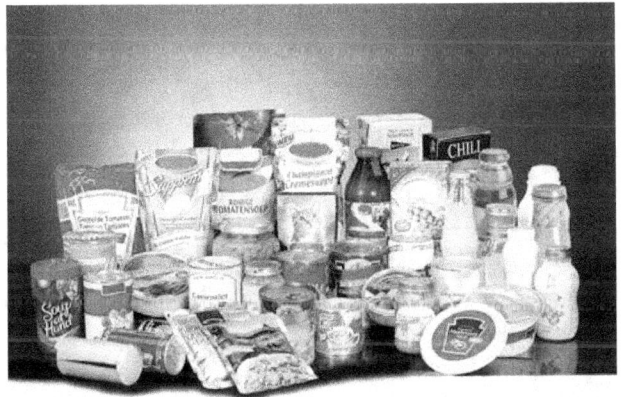

The "vegan food is healthy food" perception

A lot of starting vegans have the impression that all vegan foods are healthy.

While it's true that most processed foods like veggie hot dogs and burgers are vegan, they are heavily altered, loaded with sodium, fat and other chemicals while being stripped of their natural nutrients.

Yes, they came from plants but there is almost nothing left from the antioxidants, fibre, and other beneficial compounds they were inside before they were processed.

Diet experts discourage clients to switch to a vegan diet if they will only rely on heavily processed vegan foods.

If you want to be a successful vegan, **consume primarily real, fresh, whole and unprocessed foods.**

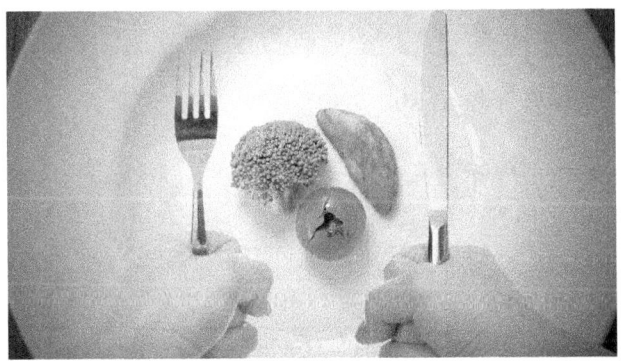

Inadequate food intake

Do you always feel hungry on your new diet?

If you do, then you are not eating enough.

Two of the biggest differences between vegan and non-vegan foods are their **caloric density and digestibility**.

Meat-based diets are high in calories and harder to digest while vegan diets are low in calories and easier to digest.

Now that your diet is composed of plant-based foods, you have to consume larger quantities to satisfy your body's needs.

Experts recommend eating natural and whole foods whenever you feel hunger, and at the same time wholesome and unprocessed.

Just because your body craves a certain food does not mean your body NEEDS it.

What it means is your body is in need of or lacking certain nutrients. With the help of your doctor, reassess your diet plan right away.

Always bring healthy snacks so you will have something to eat in between meals.

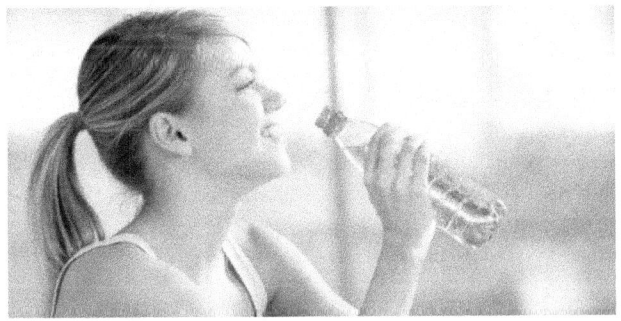

Low water intake

Another mistake new vegans make is not drinking enough water.

Now that you're on a vegan diet, you body is getting more fibre from the food you eat which mainly consists of vegetables, fruits and legumes.

Drinking 8 glasses of water or more promotes regular bowel movement through efficient handling of dietary fibre in the body.

Eat water-laden foods like cucumber and watermelon for better digestion. Otherwise, you will eventually feel discomfort in your bowel movement.

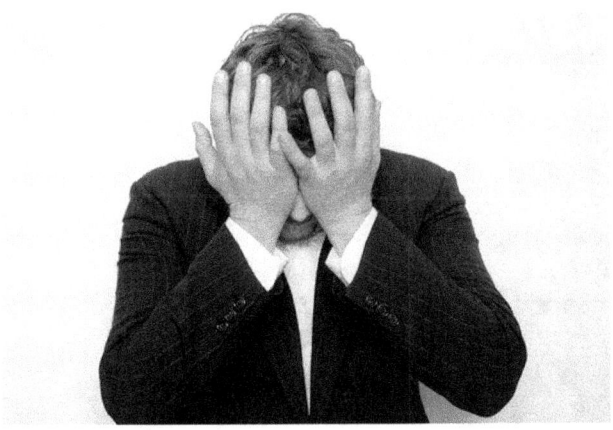

Giving up too early

After you have finally decided to do switch, you will face a lot of challenges and criti- cisms.

You may have a lot of difficulty planning your weekly diet plan due to lack of knowl- edge on where to buy vegan products.

Some people may question your reasons for doing the switch, even your family.

Do not give up. Everything you are experiencing is just normal.

The food you eat might make you feel strange or uncomfortable. No need to worry as your body is just adjusting to your new diet which usually takes 3 to 4 weeks.

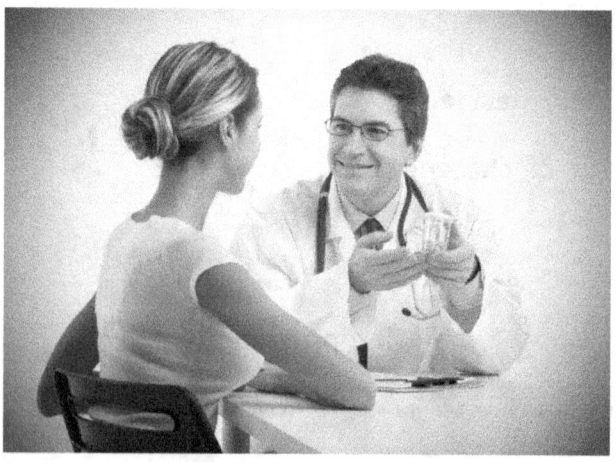

Not telling your doctor about it

Your body's needs are different from everyone else's.

Therefore, it is important that you tell your doctor about your new diet, especially when you are taking medications for a medical condition.

Your doctor will shed light on the things you don't know about veganism.

Talking to a dietician or a nutritionist is also a great help not only in determining the nutrients your body needs, but also in planning of your everyday meals for a nutritionally-balanced diet.

Overall, the best tip for all new vegans is to plan.

The vegan lifestyle has a lot of positive health benefits, but only if it is well-planned and filled with fruits, vegetables, whole grains, and heart-healthy fats.

A well-planned vegan diet and great effort to avoid the mistakes above is sure to lead you to a successful vegan lifestyle.

BONUS TIME: If you care about animals…

Mariann Sullivan and Jasmin Singer run ourhenhouse.org whose stated goal is to "effectively mainstream the movement to end the exploitation of animals".

These two hardworking women run a full blog dedicated to that mission along with 2 fantastic podcasts and one television show.

Check them out - they are one of my favourite destinations on the web.

Eggplant, Pesto and Mushroom Pizza with Tofu

Who said vegans are not allowed to eat pizza?

Of course, we have our own version of pizza, just as yummy but only healthier.

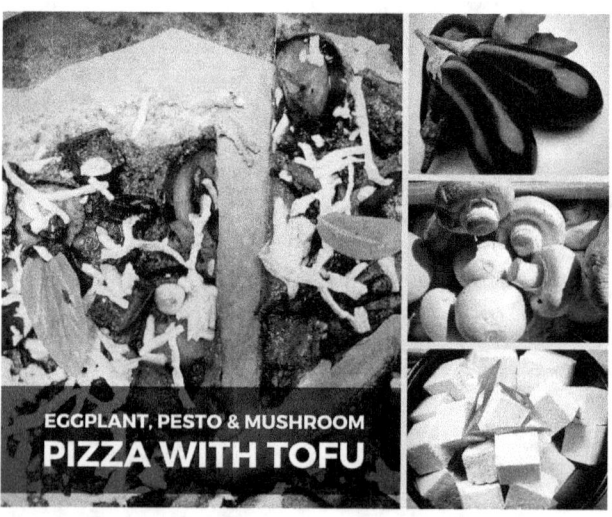

Crust

If you want to make your own gluten free crust, prepare the following:

- 2 1/4 cups all purpose flour

- 1/2 teaspoon sugar

- 1 packet yeast

- 2 tablespoons olive oil

- 3/4 to 1 cup warm water

- 2 teaspoons sea salt & pepper

- dried herbs of your choice

Pesto

- 1 cup tightly packed fresh basil leaves

- 1/3 cup pine nuts

- 5-6 olives

- 3 cloves garlic

- 1 tablespoon olive oil

- salt & pepper, to taste

- vegan milk, as needed

Toppings

- 1 small eggplant

- 4-5 mushrooms

- 5 cloves garlic, sliced thin

- 1/2 package tofu

- 2 tablespoons tamari

- 2 tablespoons olive oil

- 2 tablespoons maple syrup

- salt & pepper

Preparation

Crust

Run the outside of your mixing bowl into very warm water then combine the yeast and warm water in it.

Sprinkle little sugar to feed the yeast. Let it rise for about 10 minutes.

Add olive oil, salt, pepper and your chosen dried herbs. I suggest thyme, rosemary and basil.

Knead the dough or mix in your mixer for 8 to 10 minutes until it's soft and elastic.

Wait until it doubles in size (around 1 hour.)

Roll it out into a pizza crust. Partially bake it for 8-10 minutes at 425 degrees.

Pesto

In your food processor, blend all ingredients until spreadable and delicious.

Spread it on your partially-baked crust.

Gather all the ingredients for toppings. Sauté the tofu and garlic slices in 1 table-spoon each of olive oil, Tamari, and maple syrup.

Cook until brown.

Then, slice thinly the eggplant and mush-rooms and rub in the remaining Tamari, olive oil, and maple syrup.

Add a dash of salt, pepper and other spices you wish to add.

Add the cooked tofu to the eggplant and mushrooms.

Let it marinate until your pizza is ready.

--

Want to print this recipe? <u>Click here</u>

BONUS TIME: Meet Nava Atlas

Nava Atlas is a real pioneer in the vegan land.

She's been a featured author on big vegan blogs like Vegetarian Times, VegNews.com and Cooking Light among others.

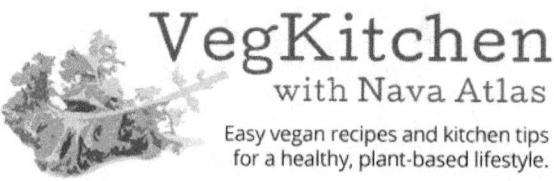

On top of that Nava has several best-selling books on vegan and vegetarian eating that you MUST check out.

For more details be sure to check out her website vegkitchen.com which is a treasure trove of recipes, advice and facts on nutrition for vegans.

Optimal Cooking Temperatures for Vegan Food

Enzymes are very important components of our food.

They are responsible for the body's use of nutrients, aid in digestion process, and keep us away from many diseases.

What we don't know is, when we cook food we can reduce or destroy the enzymes and nutrients in them.

With that said, you might be thinking raw foods (not heated above 118°F) are better.

Well, not at all times.

Some foods may be less nutritious when raw especially when they contain enzyme inhibitors that destroy nutrients.

If not heated, these substances will prevent the enzyme from performing its proper function.

On the other hand, meat, eggs and other poultry products are naturally harmful when consumed raw or undercooked.

Temperatures that "kill" enzymes

Aside from processing food, cooking at high temperatures destroys the enzymes and nutrients that allow the food to be efficiently digested.

Therefore, before the body can make use of cooked food, it must produce enzymes to aid in the digestion process.

There are still a lot of debates on exactly which cooking temperatures are destructive but here is what the experts have to say:

- Some enzymes can withstand temperatures other enzymes can't.

- Prolonged exposure to temperatures over 118°F will destroy enzymes.

- Most enzymes die at around 140°F to 158°F in a wet state.

- All enzymes are destroyed at a dry-heat temperature of about 150°F.

- All minerals retain the same amount under any temperature.

Dehydrating food and low-temp cooking

Some raw foodies and vegans practice food dehydration and low-temperature cooking to retain enzymes in food.

Here are the things you need to keep in mind about these processes:

- Dehydration is done not only to lower the risk of mold and bacteria, but also to make the food withstand relatively higher temperatures.

- There is a difference between air temperature and food temperature. The thermostat in your dehydrator regulates the air temperature.

- When dehydrating food, start at a higher temperature then reduce to a lower temp after two hours. (Example: 120°F to 105°F)

- Moist food is approximately 20 degrees cooler than the dehydrator's air temperature.

- Only wet foods are vulnerable to enzyme destruction.

- If food is dried, its enzymes can withstand

temperatures of up to 150°F without getting destroyed.

Enzymes are so powerful that they can still be able to sprout after hours of dehydration.

Try it yourself and be amazed.

Effect of diminishing enzymes

Diminishing enzymes has become a topic of concern as more and more processed and refined food products invade our diet.

Meanwhile, diseases continue to rise in number and incidence.

The more fat, sugar and starch you eat, the less likely your body's enzymes will function.

Aside from that, you may also experience bloating, fatigue and stress due to indigestion.

Enzymes from plant-based foods aid in fast and efficient digestion.

They hasten the extraction of nutrients, which in turn results to quick elimination of food from the body.

This way, the body gets rid of toxins real fast to keep the body in the best of health.

To ensure an enzyme-rich diet, try steaming rather than boiling, or broil rather than fry.

You can also eat your food warm or cool to keep the enzymes.

These ways can significantly reduce the loss of nutrients from food and harvest the health benefits enzymes bring about.

Wild Rice Salad

If you prefer rice that is grain-free and gluten-free, wild rice is the perfect option for you.

This wild rice recipe only takes 5 minutes to prepare, making 4 to 6 servings.

Each 130-kcalorie serving has 4g protein and 4g fibre.

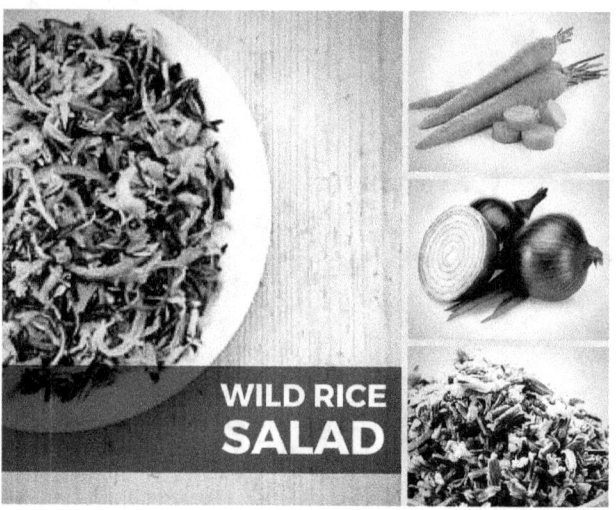

WILD RICE
SALAD

Ingredients

- 250g wild rice (microwaveable)

- 1 small handful of sultanas

- 3 carrots, grated

- 1 red onion, sliced thin-

  ly

- 1 lemon, zested and

  juiced

- 1 tbsp of honey

- Preparation

Heat the wild rice. Follow the pack's instruction.

Put the sultanas and sliced onions and in a bowl and pour boiling water on them.

After a minute, drain water and add the wild rice and carrot.

Stir the mixture.

Sprinkle the lemon zest and juice, and then drizzle honey and seasoning.

Happy eating!

--

Want to print this recipe? <u>Click here</u>

What Foods to Freeze / Leave Out / Refrigerate

Now that you are a vegan, a large part of your shopping trip will be perishable goods.

As vegans, we want our food to be as fresh as possible so knowledge on shelf life of our groceries is very important.

To avoid the wasting of resources, here is a helpful summary of the recommended storage conditions and some tips that may help prevent early spoilage or decay.

Flour: Cool, dry place; pantry (3-6 months)
- Store in glass jars to prevent moisture.

Nuts: Cool, dry place; pantry (6 months) - Store in glass jars to prevent moisture.

Seeds: Cool, dry place; pantry (2-3 years) - May be stored in the freezer for longer shelf life

Beans: Cool, dry place; pantry (6 months to 1 year) - Store in sealed glass jars. Don't put them in the freezer.

Whole Grains: Cool, dry place; pantry (Intact whole grain: 4-8 months, whole grain flour/meal: 1-3 months) - Use airtight containers to maintain freshness and will keep the grains from absorbing moisture, odours and flavours from other foods.

Tofu: Fridge (4-5 days), freezer (6-8 weeks) - Remove from original packaging and rewrap tightly when freezing.

Herbs: Fridge (3-4 days) - Place delicate herbs in plastic, secure with a rubber band, and refrigerate. You may also freeze and preserve fresh herbs in olive oil.

Avocados, Bananas, Citrus, Kiwi, Melons, Pears, Peaches, Pineapple: Room temperature or cool pantry (2-4 days) - Don't slice unless you're ready to consume it, unless you're freezing the lot.

Apples, Berries, Cherries, Grapes, Cucumber: Fridge (4-6 days) - Get rid of the ones showing signs of decay.

Artichokes: Fridge (1 week) - Sprinkle some water and store in a plastic bag.

Carrots: Fridge (1-3 months) - Store in a perforated (holes in it) plastic bag.

Kale: Fridge (7-10 days) - Remove moisture. Store in a perforated plastic bag.

Leeks, Peppers, Turnips: Fridge (1 week) - Do not wash. Store in a perforated paper bag.

Ripe Tomatoes: Room temperature (1 week) - Keep the stems during storage.

Mushrooms: Fridge (7-10 days) - Put them on a single-layer tray or in an unclosed paper bag.

Potatoes (Sweet & Plain): Dark, cool, moist area (2-4 months) - Place in a box. Make sure the location is well-ventilated.

Spinach: Fridge (2-3 days) - Wrap in paper towels and store in a plastic bag.

Leafy Greens (Celery, Broccoli, Lettuce): Fridge (4-5 weeks) - Wrap in tin foil before storing in the fridge.

Onions & Garlic: Cool dry and dark place; pantry (2-3 months) - Place in a perforated paper bag. Keep away from potatoes as they promote spoilage of each other.

Smoky Maple Homemade Seitan Sandwich

Seitan is a vegetarian meat substitute that is a great source of protein. Unlike tofu and tempeh, this one is different for its meaty texture.

When you eat seitan, it feels like you're chewing actual meat.

In order for you to know seitan better, here is a single-serving hearty sandwich recipe that will surely make your meat-eating friends drool.

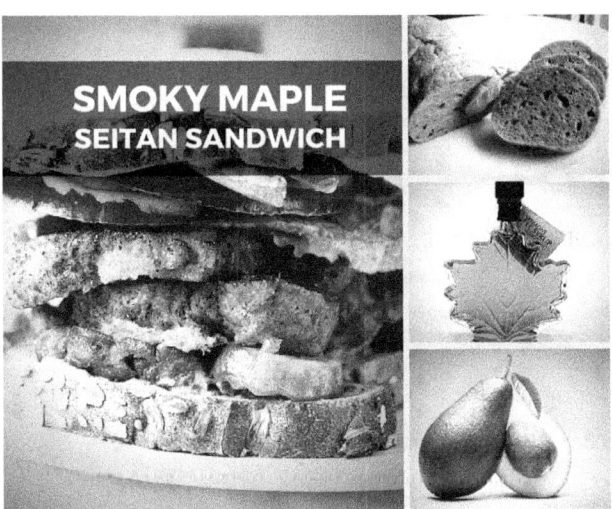

SMOKY MAPLE
SEITAN SANDWICH

Ingredients for Seitan

- 4 slices pepper mushroom seitan, about 1/2 inch thick

- 1-3 tsp maple syrup

- 1 tsp liquid smoke

- 1-4 tsp olive oil

- fine black pepper, to taste

- salt or tamari, to taste

Preparation

Heat olive oil in a frying pan and sauté the seitan. Add the maple syrup, fine black pepper and liquid smoke. Cook each side for about 2 minutes until seitan is heated through and crispy browned edges form. Let it cool for a few minutes. Proceed to next step.

Ingredients for Sandwich

- cooked seitan

- 2 slices multi-grain bread, toasted

- 3 leaves romaine

- 2 thin red onion slices

- 3 thin slices avocado

- 2-3 pickles

- 2 tsp Dijon mustard

- 2 tsp Vegenaise

- 1 tsp chipotle hot sauce

- fine black pepper, to taste

- Preparation

Toast the bread.

Spread Dijon mustard on one slice and Veg-enaise and chipotle mixture on the other.

Put seitan on top of one bread.

Stack the onion, romaine, avocado, pepper and pickles.

Put the other bread on top.

Slice the stacked sandwich then serve.

--

Want to print this recipe? Click here

Fake Meat Showdown

With the continuously growing awareness on veganism, more and more meat substitutes enter the market today.

You will be surprised how many varieties are already available in grocery stores around you.

For new vegans, meat substitutes aka fake meat aka mock meat can be helpful in their transition process into full-fledged vegans.

Some, however, refuse to try these kinds of meat. They would rather make them themselves. They have their reasons.

To help you decide which to buy, here is a list of ten vegan meats and some helpful tips about them:

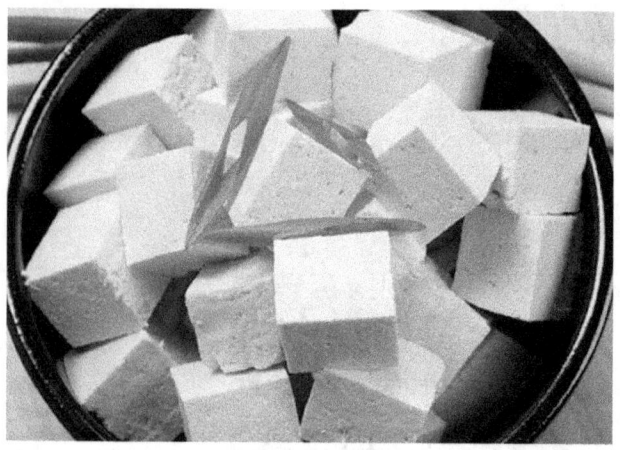

Tofu

I'm sure that before you started your vegan diet, your research has already proved the versatility of tofu in the diet.

As mentioned earlier in this book, it can be added to practically any dish. So, I know this will most likely be your top meat substitute.

It's simple, cheap and easy to prepare. Plus, it can be also used as a dessert. Just make sure it is well-drained and well-pressed before cooking.

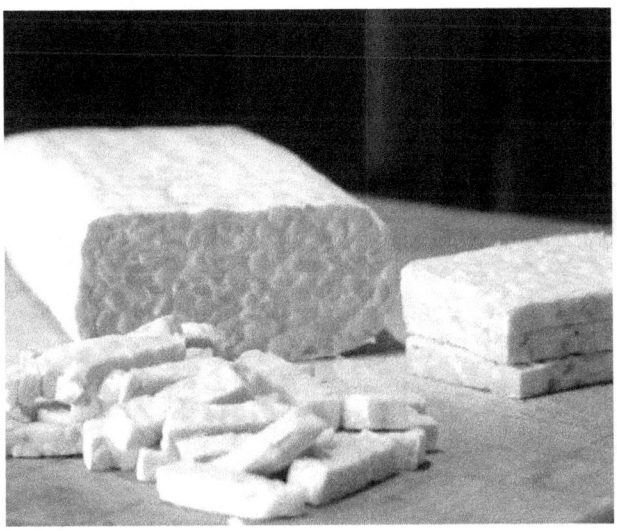

Tempeh

Tempeh is very much like tofu, as it is also derived from soy.

The main difference would be the preparation: it undergoes fermentation.

Nutrition-wise, it is a very good homemade vegan meat product as it contains more than **twice the protein content of tofu.**

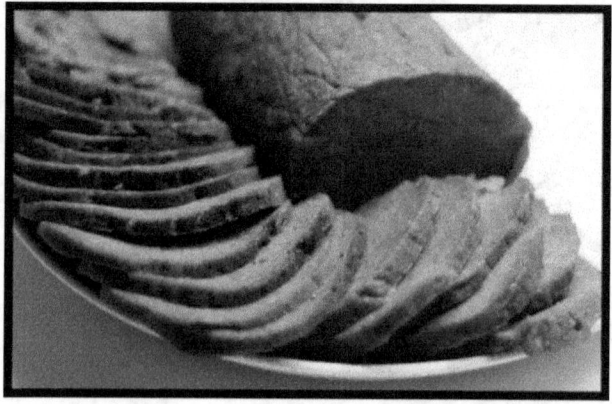

Seitan

Vegans use seitan more than any other meat substitute when it comes to DIY recipes. Like tofu and tempeh, you can be experimental when preparing it.

You can use whatever kind of flavour you want. It looks and feels like real meat. Seitan is made from wheat flour.

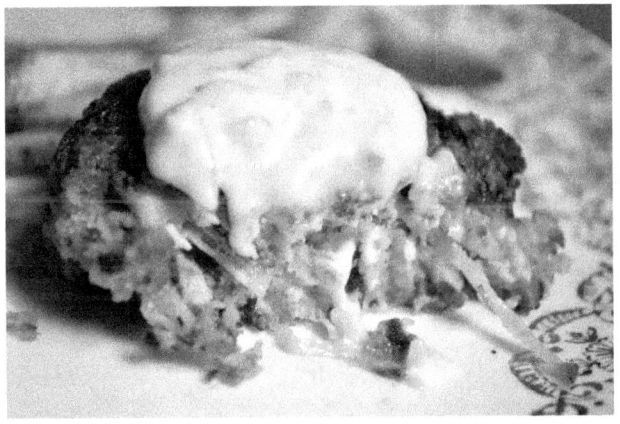

Vegan Crab Cakes

If you are not into the soy-derived meats, then you can try making your own vegan crab cakes. It is a mixture of hearts of palm and a variety of seasonings.

However, this requires a lot of time and effort to make as there is only a few pre-processed versions of these in the market.

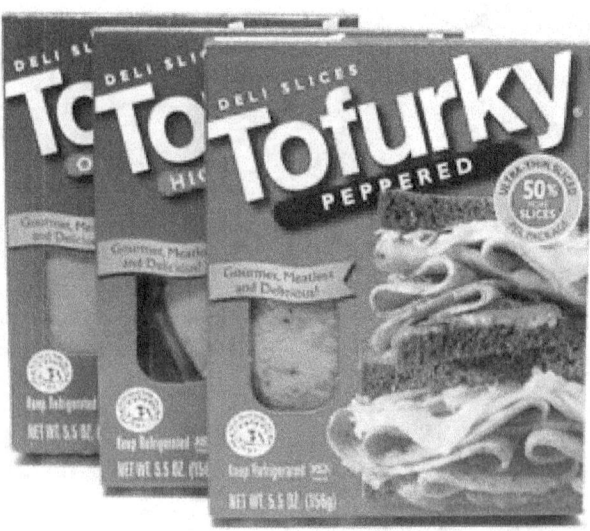

Tofurky Deli Slices

Tofurky deli slices offer a wide variety of tasty fake meat made from smoked wheat gluten.

Some flavours of their products are pepperoni, smoked-ham and bologna.

Although these meats are vegan, they are processed so health benefits may be greatly reduced.

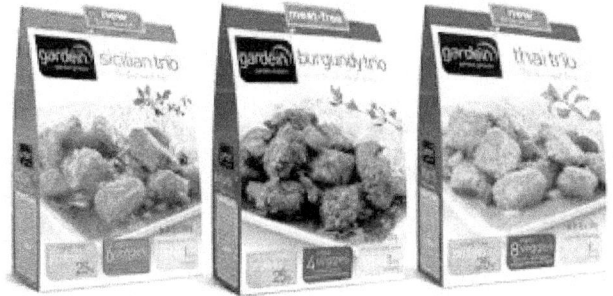

Gardein products

Gardein offers a number of faux chicken, pork, beef, turkey and fish products, mostly gourmet.

They also have gluten-free meats and pock-et meals for you convenience.

However, like Tofurky, these are all pro-cessed products.

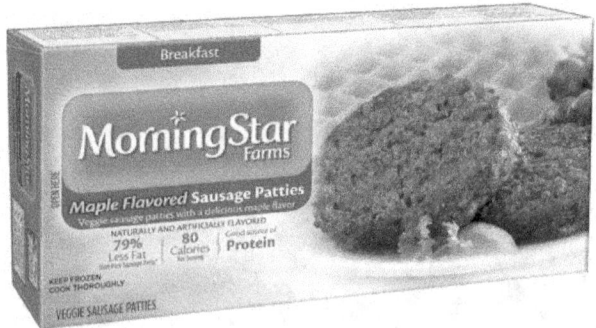

Morningstar Farms sausage patties with maple syrup

Both Tofurky and Gardein are loved for their tasty meats, but the maple syrup in Morningstar Farms sausage patties made the difference.

You will find this brand in almost every grocery store in your neighbourhood.

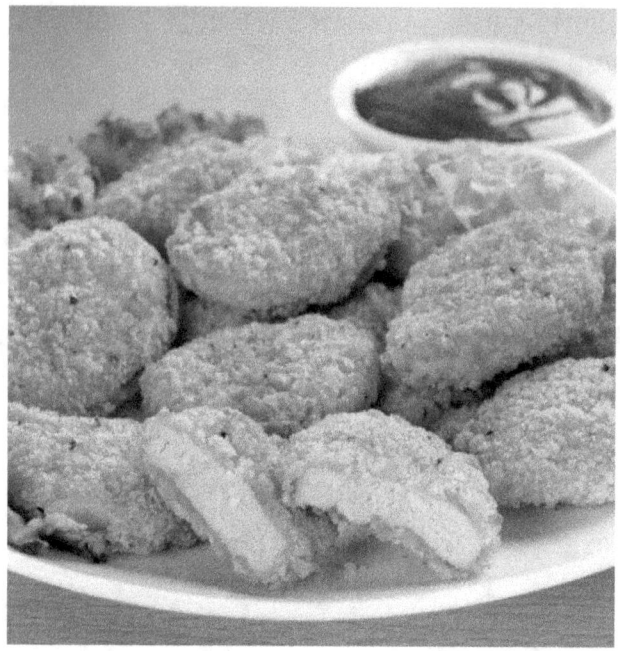

Quorn Chicken nuggets

These vegetarian chicken nuggets are known for its excellent imitation of chicken meat's taste and texture. But it turns out that these contain eggs so they are not intended for vegan consumption.

Mei Wah Drumsticks

Like Quorn, Mei Wah also produces vegetarian chicken meat, only in drumstick form. They can be baked or fried just like normal chicken meat; and they come with a wooden dowel substituting the chicken bone.

Sunshine Veg Kebab

A bestseller of the Sunshine brand, the Veg Kebab is famous for having an appearance, texture and flavour almost identical to real beef that can be used for different dishes. Sunshine brand, just like the other five in this list, produce processed meats.

There are a lot of vegetarian meats available in the market, and aside from the fake meats mentioned above, the list continues to go on.

Many vegetarian meats may be vegan, but some contain traces of egg and other dairy products. So, if you are planning to buy items on this list, make sure you read the label. Experts still recommend eating whole over processed food for maximum health benefits.

BONUS: Keep up with Vegan News

If you want the latest in vegan news then check out LatestVeganNews.com (perfect name am I right).

Hannah Sentence curated and produces some of the best news coming out for vegans.

LATEST VEGAN NEWS

Check out her website and join a passionate community of fellow activists.

Red Lentil Soup

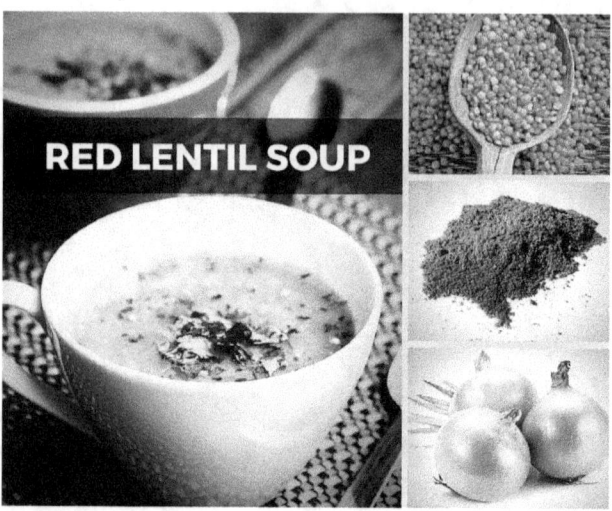

Ingredients

- 1 cup red lentils, washed and soaked in water for 1 hr

- ½ - 1 teaspoon cumin

- ½ -1 teaspoon garam masala

- ½ - 1 teaspoon smoked paprika

- 1 tablespoon extra virgin olive oil

- 1-2 teaspoons minced ginger

- 2-3 cloves garlic, minced

- 1 onion, diced

- 1 teaspoon salt

- 4 cups vegetable broth

- 1 cup water

For garnish: red pepper flakes, lime juice, fresh cilantro, chopped

Preparation

Heat oil in a pot over medium heat. Add onion. Cook until translucent. Add ginger and cook for 1 minute.

Add garlic and cook for 1 minute. Stir occasionally.

Add cumin, garam masala, smoked paprika and salt. Mix well.

Add red lentils, broth and water. Bring to a boil then reduce heat. Let it simmer covered for 30 minutes or until lentils cooked.

Puree with immersion blender if creamy texture is desired.

Serve sprinkled with red pepper flakes, a squeeze of lime juice and teaspoon of fresh cilantro, chopped.

--

Want to print this recipe? Click here

Meet Your New Weekly (Monthly) Shopping List

Don't know what to stock for the month?

Trips to the grocery store should never be a chore. Below, I've put together a list of items that I regularly buy at the store.

I've organized them as must-haves - which are versatile enough to be included in many salads, soups, and other dishes.

Things like sweet potatoes which can be the base for a soup while also steamed and placed in a salad.

The other group are optional items which are not as versatile and I only pickup when I have a specific dish in mind. Things like Okra which are hard to include in a salad for instance.

Without further ado, here's my list of food items to guide you on your grocery shopping (feel free to change as you like):

Vegetables

Must-haves: Avocado, Bell peppers, Broccoli, Cabbage, Carrots, Cauliflower, Celery, Corn, Cucumber, Eggplant, Garlic, Kale, Lettuce, Onions, Peas, Shallots / Leeks or Spinach, Squash, Sweet potatoes, Tomatoes

Optional: Asparagus, Beets, Brussels Sprouts, Collard Greens, Ginger, Hot peppers, Mushrooms, Okra, Radishes, Taro, Turnips /

Parsnips, Water Chestnuts, Watercress, Zucchini

Grains

Must-haves: Brown rice, Oatmeal, Quinoa, Wild rice

Optional: Amaranth, Barley, Buckwheat, Couscous

Nuts / Beans

Must-haves: Black beans, Chickpeas, Kidney beans, Lentils, Mung beans, Pinto beans, Almonds, Walnuts, Cashews

Optional: Black-eyed peas, Lima beans, Red beans, White beans

Oils / Spices

Must-haves: Olive oil, Coconut oil, Basil, Black pepper, Cilantro, Cumin, Curry powder, Garlic, Nutmeg, Parsley, Peppermint, Rosemary, Vanilla extract

Optional: Sesame oil, Cayenne pepper, Chilli powder, Dill, Lemongrass, Oregano, Paprika, Red pepper, Thyme, Turmeric

Meat Substitutes

Must-haves: Tofu, Tempeh

Optional: Seitan

Liquids

Must-haves: Almond milk, Coconut water

Optional: Soy milk, Rice milk

Powders

Must-haves: Nutritional yeast, Protein powders

Optional: Cacao powder, Acai powder

Sweeteners

Must-haves: Agave nectar

Optional: Maple syrup, Stevia

Dairy and Cheese Substitutes

Must-haves: Almond butter

Optional: Soy butter, Soy creamer, Soy margarine

Condiments

Must-haves: Salsa, Hummus, Soy sauce, Sriracha, Mustard, Balsamic Vinegar

Optional: Vegan mayo, Vegetable bouillon

Leek, Artichoke & Lentil Mung Bean Linguine

Here's a protein-packed, gluten-free pasta substitute that delivers an astounding 20g of protein for every 187-calorie serving!

Leeks, artichokes and lentils are high in protein and provide a wonderful, filling mix of flavours.

This dish is even topped with cheesy nutritional yeast which is rich in Vitamin B12.

You are sure to receive plenty of health benefits from this 4-serving hearty meal.

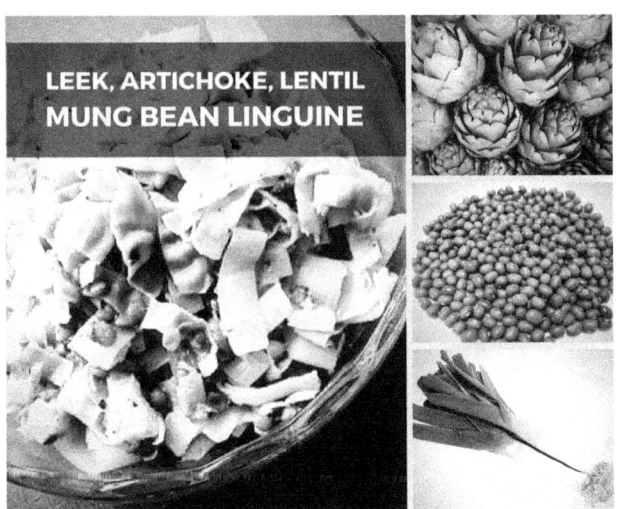

LEEK, ARTICHOKE, LENTIL MUNG BEAN LINGUINE

Ingredients

- 1 package (7.05oz) organic mung bean linguine

- 2 medium leeks (white and light green parts only), chopped

- 1 12oz can artichoke hearts, sliced

- 1 can organic lentils

- Juice of 1 lemon

- 1 clove garlic, diced

- ½ yellow onion, diced

- ½ cup vegan nutritional yeast

- 1 Tbsp vegan margarine

- Salt and pepper to taste

Preparation

1. Heat the margarine in a pot over medium-low heat.

2. Add the garlic, onion, and leeks, and cook until caramelized.

3. Add the artichokes and sauté for about 3 minutes. Next, put in the lentils and lemon. Sprinkle some salt and pepper to taste.

4. Turn heat to low, cover and let it simmer for 5-10 minutes.

5. Cook the mung bean linguine per the package instructions and reserve 1/2 cup of pasta water.

6. Add the cooked mung bean linguine into the pot with the artichoke/ lentil mixture.

7. Add the nutritional yeast and reserved pasta water as needed.

8. Mix well. Add fresh lemon juice for a citrusy twist.

--

Want to print this recipe? <u>Click here</u>

Stop Asking: We Get Enough Protein…Let Me Explain

Most critics of veganism challenge the ability for this diet to provide enough protein.

They spread inaccurate and sometimes unsubstantiated claims about protein content in vegetables and other plant-based food.

Here are four myths about the vegan diet busted:

Myth: Vegetables don't have enough protein.

Fact: **We only need 2.5% to 11% of our calories from protein** according to the WHO and this includes safety margins for people who need more protein than the average person.

Vegetables can provide more than enough of that protein.

Critics don't seem to understand that each and every whole plant-based food contains more than 2.5% protein.

In fact, nuts, seeds, grains and vegetables average at least 11 percent protein content (fruits sit at 6.7%).

So you can get protein from eating any whole plant-based food as LONG as you're eating ENOUGH.

Myth: Plant protein has poor quality.

Fact: Studies show that plant-based protein can provide the full range of amino acids your body requires.

The body doesn't necessarily care about the protein's quality as much as it does the adequacy of your protein intake, regardless of the source.

Critics boast meat's higher protein amounts.

But does it make the body healthy? NO!

Experts say a very large amount of protein intake is harmful to your health.

Overconsumption of protein has been linked to problems like bone loss, osteoporosis, renal diseases and cancer growth.

Myth: Vegetables are harder to digest than meat.

Fact: The digestibility of protein in beef and fish may be impressively high at 94 percent, but plant-based foods such as peanut butter and flour have even higher digestibility rates of 95 and 96 percent, respectively.

Corn, rice, oatmeal and peas may have lower digestibility rate of 86 to 88 percent but the difference is insignificant.

Myth: You can't be a bodybuilder when you're vegan.

Fact: Yes you can! As long as you do regular weight training and eat enough diverse fruits, vegetables and other plant-based foods that are rich in protein, you can definitely maintain or build your body muscles.

A vegan diet can deliver not only the protein needs of the body, but also its other nutritional needs like vitamins, macronutrients, etc. to help you sustain a healthy lifestyle.

—-

For more information and the source of all this data, check out the following links:

163

- <u>Setting the Record Straight about Protein</u>

- <u>10 Myths About Vegetarian Diets</u>

First Rule of the Veggie Club

Enjoy this tasty and colourful sandwich with just 10-minutes prep time.

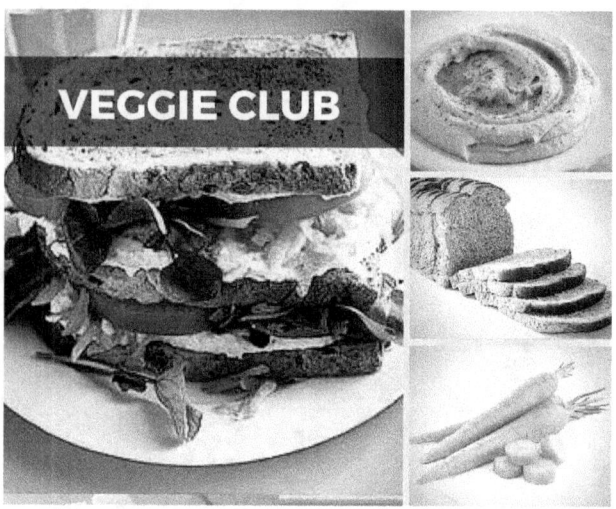

Ingredients

-   3 slices bread

- 2 tomatoes, thickly sliced

- I large handful water-cress

- I carrot, peeled and coarsely grated

- I ½ tbsp hummus

- I small squeeze lemon juice

- I tbsp olive oil

Preparation

Toast the bread.

In a bowl, mix the watercress, carrots, olive oil and lemon juice.

Then, spread hummus on one side of each toasted bread.

One 1 slice, put some watercress and carrot mixture. Then, top that with another slice.

Lay some tomatoes. Close the sandwich with the last toasted bread, hummus side down.

Eat and enjoy!

--

Want to print this recipe? Click here

Do Vegans Need to Take Supplements?

Everyone needs regular and dependable sources of B12 especially vegans and people over the age of 50 following any kind of diet.

Of the two groups, vegans are the ones who are more susceptible of being Vitamin B12 deficient as the vitamin has no plant source.

If not taken seriously, very low B12 intake can cause anemia and nerve damage.

Sources

Vitamin B12 generally comes from microorganisms. But as mentioned above, there is no plant source of Vitamin B12.

Good thing, there are a lot of vegan food items available in the market today that are fortified with vitamin B12.

Some of them are in milks, yogurts, spreads, breakfast cereals, and nutritional yeast products.

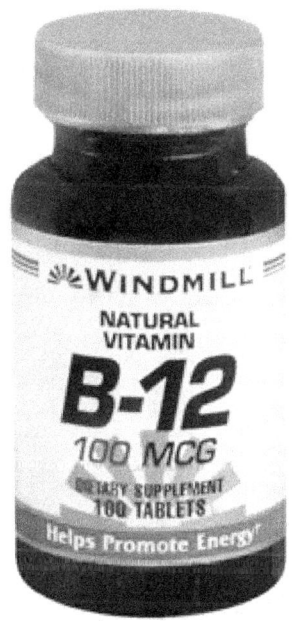

The other B12 source are smart supplements that you can take daily or weekly to give you enough amounts of B12 to be absorbed by the body.

Vitamin B12 should be taken in small amounts, but as often as possible. Therefore, if you don't get to have B12 often, you need to take more of it.

For many decades, studies have proven that B12 fortified foods and supplements are the only reliable sources of Vitamin B12 for vegans.

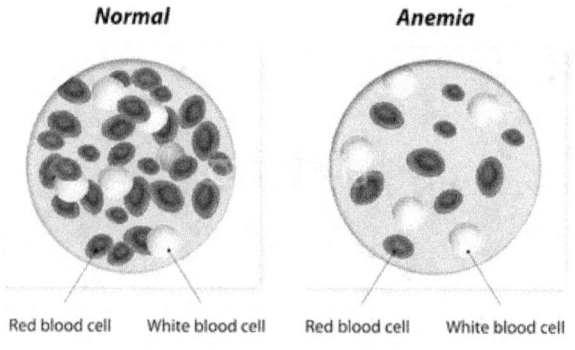

Normal   Anemia

Red blood cell   White blood cell   Red blood cell   White blood cell

Symptoms of B12 deficiency

Symptoms of deficiency differ from person to person but it usually takes five years or more to develop in adults.

For some, they experience problems in just a period as short as a year. Here are some symptoms you should watch out for:

- strange sensations, numbness, or tingling in the hands, legs, or feet

- difficulty in walking

- weakness or fatigue

- yellowed skin or jaundice

- anemia

- a swollen, inflamed tongue

- difficulty thinking and reasoning or memory loss

- paranoia or hallucinations

Very low B12 intake can lead to neurologic problems, blood diseases, potential risk of heart disease and elevated homocysteine levels.

B12 deficiency also affects pregnant women and their babies. It is linked to the baby's loss of appetite and energy. Sometimes, it can lead to a coma or death.

Recommendations

The US recommended intake is 2.4 micrograms a day for ordinary adults and 2.8 micrograms for pregnant women or nursing mothers.

The absorption rate of B12 is around 50 percent so if you are taking 2.4 micrograms per day, your body absorbs around 1.2 micrograms daily.

Doctors recommend three ways to get Vitamin B12:

- Incorporate fortified foods to each meal to get 3 micrograms of vitamin B12 every day.

- Take one 10-microgram supplement of vitamin B12 every day.

- Take one 2000-microgram supplement of vitamin B12 every week.

As a general reminder, talk to your doctor about Vitamin B12. Always check nutrition labels and details so you can keep track of your B12 intake.

More importantly, know what you are eating. A well-informed vegan will have no problem with B12 intake.

—-

Want to learn more check out the sources of all this great information:

- What Every Vegan Should Know about Vitamin B12

- Vitamin B12 : your key facts

- Vitamin B12 deficiency can be sneaky, harmful

Mushroom Stroganoff

There are times when you get so busy absorbed in your daily responsibilities. But when it comes to fuelling up again to get through the day, you tend to neglect the nutrition you need.

You end up consuming processed foods, thinking they would be much easier to prepare.

Here is a quick delicious meal done in just 15 minutes. This recipe makes two servings with less than 200 calories each.

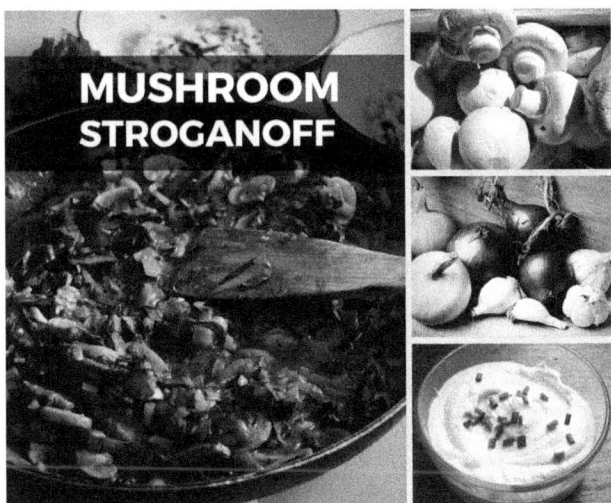

Ingredients

- 500 g mushrooms, sliced or diced

- 4 cloves garlic, minced

- I medium onion, diced

- 4 tbsp fresh parsley, chopped

- 1 tsp smoked paprika

- 50 ml vegetable stock

- 3 tbsp vegan sour cream

- 2 cups wild rice

- black pepper

Preparation

1. Heat the oil in a large frying pan over medium heat.

2. Add the onion, garlic and mushrooms. Cook for 5-10 minutes until

the onions are translu-
cent and mushrooms
are golden

3.   Add the smoked paprika and vegetable stock,
and a generous amount
of black pepper. Cook
for 5 minutes more.

4.   Put in the sour cream
and half of the parsley
into the mixture and
stir.

5.   Top it with the remaining parsley and serve
alongside wild rice.

--

Want to print this recipe? <u>Click here</u>

How do you Main Muscle Mass on a Vegan Diet?

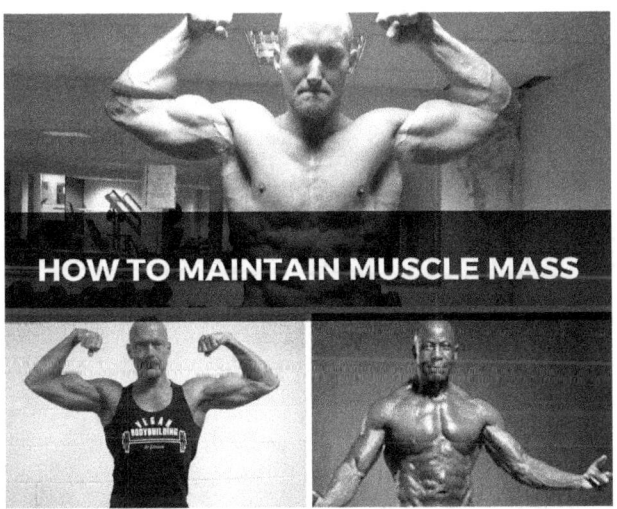

Vegans are less likely to be associated with muscles and bodybuilding. Usually, when we think of the word "vegan," we imagine a person that is skinny.

What most people don't know is vegans are equally capable of building and maintaining body muscles even in the absence of meat.

Decline in muscle mass over the years is very common especially if you do not practice weight-training.

Also, as you grow older, your body uses protein less efficiently, leading to muscle decline.

But clearly, it can also be attributed to other factors like diet, lifestyle and hormones.

According to the International Osteoporosis Foundation (IOF), older adults require 1 to 1.2 grams of protein per kilogram of body weight.

Vegans, too, are recommended to reach the upper range to maintain their muscles successfully.

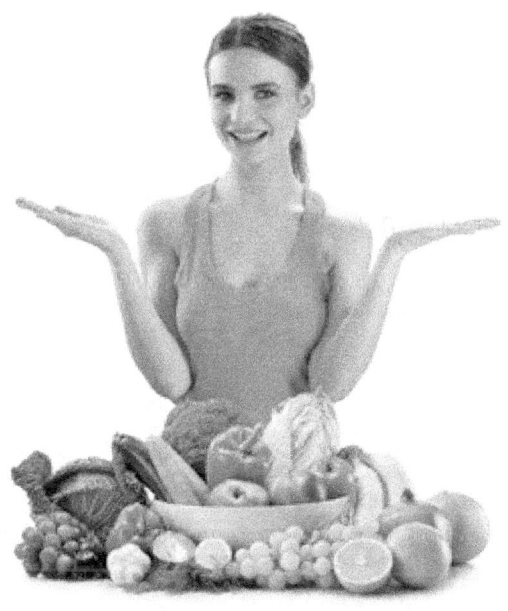

Maintain your body muscles by following these helpful tips:

1. Include weight training in your daily routine. It is the best thing you can do to build and maintain muscles.

2. Add a lot of legumes in your diet like nuts, beans and soy products. Flax and hemp seeds are great sources pro-tein and fatty acids.

3. Eat a lot of fruits and leafy green vegetables. You will reap plenty of

positive health benefits like antioxidants and folate that strengthens the muscles.

4. Look for foods that have high levels of vitamin D and B12 and incorporate them to your diet. These vitamins are linked to stronger muscles. Experts suggest at least 600 IUs of vitamin D and 25 micrograms of vitamin B12 daily.

5. Remove processed foods from your diet and replace them with whole unprocessed and nutrient-rich foods.

It is always better to prevent muscle loss than that to try to rebuild it. Therefore, while you are still young, do your best to go for better lifestyle choices.

Eat the right food and maintain an active lifestyle incorporating weight training.

By following these steps, you will be able to maintain muscle strength and tissue while on a vegan diet.

Peanut Butter Tofu Rice

This quick and healthy fibre-rich meal with a peanut buttery twist is perfect for lunch or dinner.

Feel free to add crunchy vegetables of your choice for a little flair. Top with some cilantro and chopped nuts.

Serves 2.

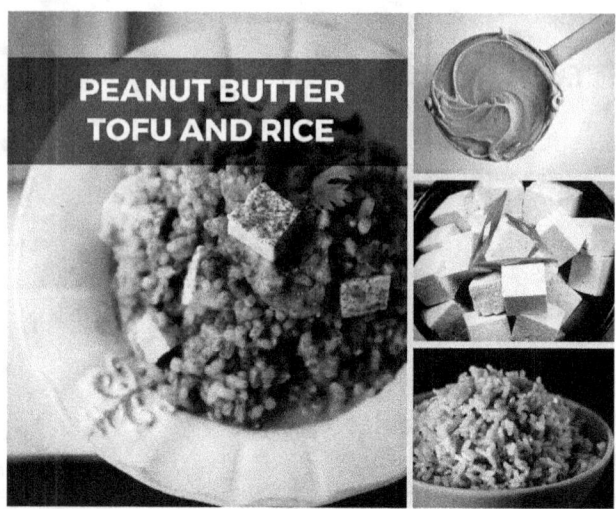

PEANUT BUTTER
TOFU AND RICE

Ingredients

- 2 1/2 cups brown rice, cooked

- 1 1/4 cups tofu, cubed

- vegetables of your choice

- chopped peanuts

- cilantro

Sauce

- 3 Tbsp peanut butter, salted / creamy

- 1 Tbsp white miso paste or lime juice

- 2-3 tsp tamari or soy sauce

- 2 1/2 tsp agave syrup

- 3/4 cup water

- 3-4 dashes cayenne powder (optional)

Preparation

Using a Vita-mix or food processor, mix and blend all the ingredients for the sauce.

Prepare your tofu. Steam or sauté them in a pan with some oil for 5-10 minutes. You can also use chilled tofu if you like.

Mix the tofu with a spoonful of the sauce.

Boil the rice and then mix it with the tofu and remaining sauce.

Add your vegetables and top it with some fresh cilantro and chopped peanuts.

Spice it up with cayenne if you like. Serve warm and enjoy!

--

Want to print this recipe? <u>Click here</u>

15 Tips for Hosting a Unforgettable Vegan Dinner Party

A new vegan hosting a dinner party?

Don't stress too much.

To have a smooth, fun and successful vegan dinner party is always possible.

Let the following tips guide you on your first time:

Create a plan

First, decide on the date and venue. Two weeks of preparation would be ideal.

List down all the important details like the number of expected guests (including kids), stuff you need to buy and what you plan cook.

Then, write a schedule of all the things you should accomplish every day until the dinner party.

Ask for your guests' suggestions

Your guests can be of great help in deciding what to include in your vegan dinner party menu.

Ask some of them to give suggestions so you'll have an idea of what they want and what they are expecting.

This way, you will also be aware if any of your guests have allergies to certain foods.

Go stationery shopping

Buy invitation cards and cards to place in front of each dish. These cards will hold the name of the dish behind it so your guests can easily identify the food and which one is their favourite.

Send out the invitations

After finalizing the plans, send out invites immediately so your guests can free the date for your dinner party.

If you are on a tight budget, you can opt for calling your guests instead rather than buying invitation cards.

Ditch the disposables

To make the event not only cruelty-free but also eco-friendly, use all of your plates, glasses, serving dishes and silverware instead of the biodegradable ones.

Don't worry if they don't match, your guests won't even remember it once they have tasted your appetizer.

Keep it simple

And by simple, I am talking about the ingredients. There is no need to use expensive ingredients especially if you're hosting a large number of guests.

With simple ingredients, you can double or triple the food's serving without spending too much.

Prepare balanced meals

Make sure to not only satisfy your guests' taste buds but also their body's nutritional needs.

Incorporate fruits, vegetables, whole grains and nuts to your meals so everyone will have a balanced intake of proteins, fats, calcium, vitamins and others.

Serve seasonal fruits and vegetables

By doing this, you will be able to save money and make the most out of your budget.

Plus, a lot of people love to eat food that is in season.

Surprise your guests with adventurous dishes

Surprise your guests by serving something they've never tasted or heard of before. Apparently there is something called fried vegan spaghetti.

Intriguing right?

Preoccupy the kids with chalk

Sidewalk chalk is a simple yet entertaining activity to have in your dinner party.

Not only that it's cheap, not permanent and biodegradable, both kids or adults can enjoy drawing or writing notes in every concrete corner of your house.

Bring your own booze

To spare yourself from having to pay for the liquor as well, ask your guests to bring their desired alcoholic drinks.

This is to avoid buying the wrong booze as many alcoholic drinks employ animal-derived materials in the process.

After all, your hands are already full with all the cooking and preparations.

Have a Non-Dairy Ice Cream or Sorbet Station

Using a Vita-mix, blend frozen fruits with unsweetened non-dairy milk. You can add cacao powder or Maca for a more flavourful dessert. Sprinkle some vegan chocolate chips for the kids to enjoy.

Invite your budding vegan friends

Now that you're a vegan, a lot of your non-vegan friends must be intrigued by your decision that they keep asking so many questions.

Invite those who show interest or openness to your new lifestyle and share with them the experience of eating cruelty-free.

Ready your party playlist

Music is the best way to liven up the mood in any kind of gathering. It creates a good atmosphere and is a good way to officially start the dinner.

Make sure though that you include many different genres so everyone can enjoy.

Vegan Peach Pie

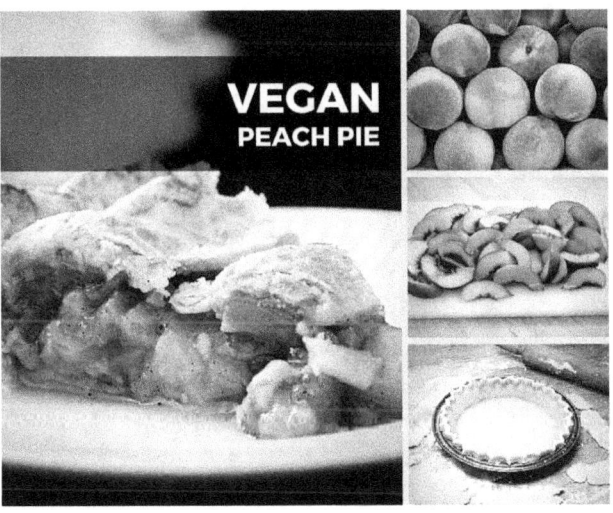

Ingredients

- 8 peaches, trimmed and sliced

- 2 vegan pie crusts

- 3 tbsp flour

- I cup brown sugar

- I tsp of cinnamon

- I tbsp of lemon juice

Preparation

In a large bowl, toss and mix the peaches, sugar, cinnamon, flour, and lemon juice. Leave for 10 minutes until the peaches are soft.

Pour the mixture on to one of the pie crusts.

Get the other crust and cut them into strips for a lattice top or you can just cover it as is. However, make sure to cut a hole

on the top crust for the steam to be re-
leased.

Bake at 350°F for 30-40 minutes until the
peaches are perfectly soft.

Serve.

--

Want to print this recipe? Click here

The Essentials Only: Kitchen Utensils for Vegans

I personally think that every vegan should learn how to cook. It is a skill you must have for your own convenience.

When I cook, I feel happy and it makes my everyday vegan diet more enjoyable.

But before you embark on your cooking adventure, you must know these three musthaves in every vegan kitchen that will make your life a whole lot easier:

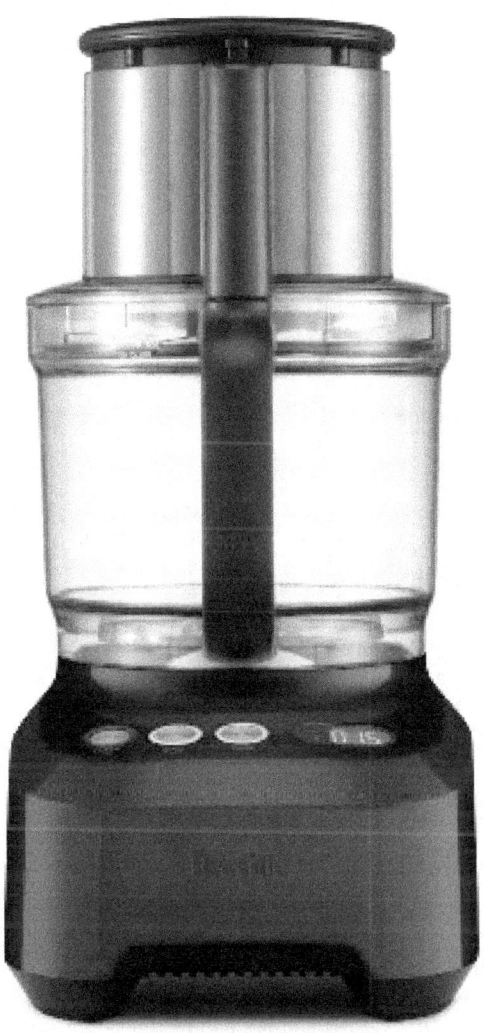

Food Processor

Cooking healthy requires fresh ingredients, but preparing your ingredients may require a lot of work.

Fortunately, a food processor exists and it can definitely save you time and energy.

Food processors are great for making soups, spreads, fillings, dips, sauces, and so much more.

I recommend the Amazon bestseller: the Breville BFP800CBXL Sous Chef food processor. comes with 5 multi-function discs and 3 blades, a 16-cup large bowl, a 2.5 cup small bowl, accessory storage and a 5.5 inch super-wide feed chute so you won't need to pre-cut most vegetables and fruits.

Truly, it is a great investment for $399.95.

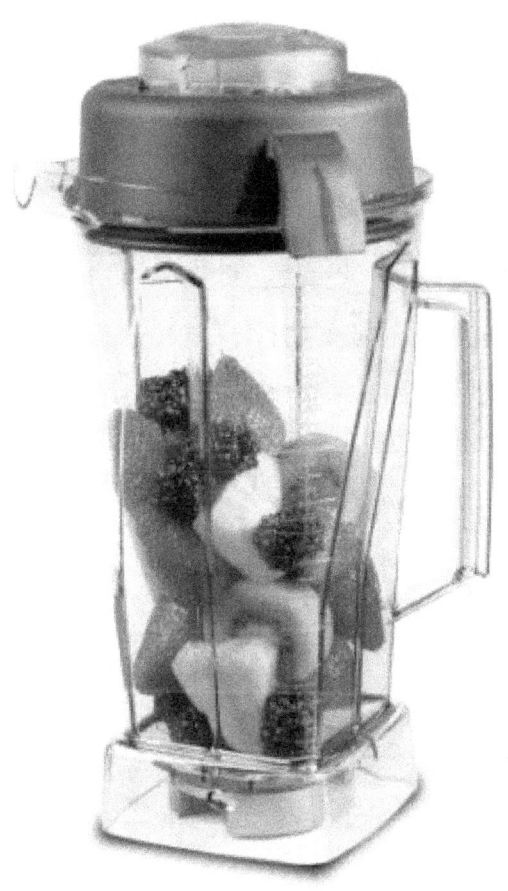

Blender

Confused to be the same as a food processor, the main function of a blender is actually to mix soft solids and liquids.

A blender is all you need in making fresh fruit smoothies, vegetable juice drinks, blended soups, sorbets, and even DIY fruity ice creams.

I recommend the $127.65 <u>Vita-mix Eastman Tritan Copolyester 64-Ounce Container with Wet Blade and Lid</u>.

Vitamix has already received notable good reviews for its high-quality blenders so you already got an assurance that this blender is reliable.

The blender is spill-proof and drip-free. The stainless steel blades are made harder and better for smooth blending.

It also allows you to transfer its content into another container without taking the lid off, just like a pitcher. More importantly, the Vita-mix is easy to clean.

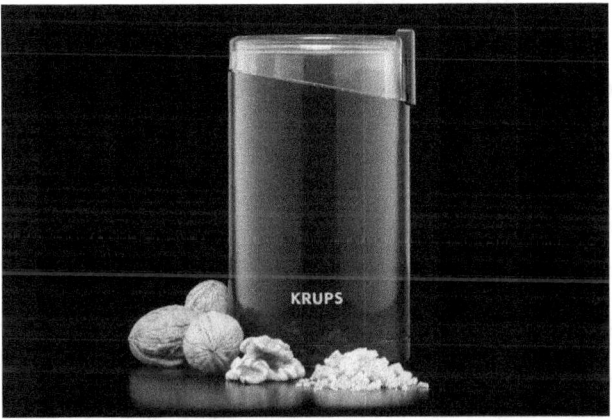

Coffee Grinder

The coffee grinder is one very interesting tool in the vegan kitchen. This amazing gizmo actually has more exciting uses aside from grinding coffee.

Ditch buying expensive flours and powders from different grains and herbs. Instead, do it yourself using your coffee grinder.

I recommend KRUPS F203 Electric Spice and Coffee Grinder.

It is a top choice for a low price of $19.99. Satisfied users report long lifespan of more than ten years, and they even use it more than once a day.

The grinder works quietly, easy to use and to control, and most importantly easy to clean (you don't want to have your coffee

tasting like your herbs and spices!)

Coconut Sugar Caramelized Plantains

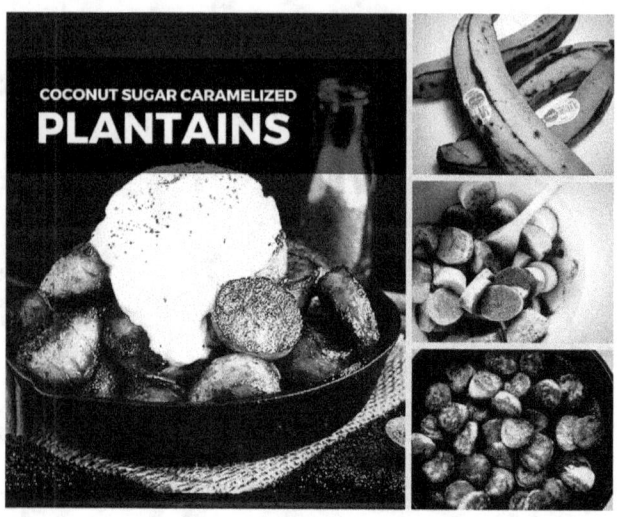

Plantains are a member of the banana family.

They look so much like a regular banana, but they longer, have thicker skin and can be in green, yellow and black colour.

Also, they are most of the time used as vegetables in the Western African and Caribbean countries.

Compared to regular bananas, plantains have more potassium, magnesium and vitamins A and C.

They are highly nutritious and can be added to a wide range of dishes.

Who knows, with only 5 ingredients and 15 minutes plantains could be your new favourite vegan dessert?

Ingredients

- 3 ripe plantains

- 3 Tbsp coconut sugar

- 1/4 tsp ground cinnamon

- 1 pinch sea salt

- 1-2 Tbsp coconut oil (or olive oil)

- Coconut whipped cream or ice cream (for topping)

Preparation

Heat a large cast iron or metal skillet over medium-high heat.

Chop your plantains into half-inch slices and mix them with coconut sugar, cinnamon and sea salt in a bowl.

Add coconut oil to the hot cast iron or skillet. Put in the sliced plantains and make sure they do not crowd.

Cook each side for 2-3 minutes until brown and caramelized.

Serve warm with coconut whipped cream or dairy free ice cream.

Keep leftovers in the fridge. They will only last for a few days.

This recipe makes 4 servings.

--

Want to print this recipe? Click here

BONUS TIME: Shout out

Shout out to this website for providing this last recipe.

If you want simple, minimal cooking check out the Minimalist Baker by John and Dana.

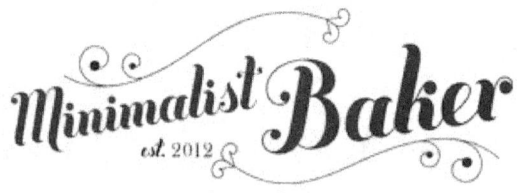

While the resources and recipes are great, where they really set themselves apart is by showing others how to launch their own food blog.

This includes a course on how to take food photography and providing readers with all the tools they used to grow and monetize their blog.

Definitely one to check out!

How to Ripen a Banana in ONLY 20 Minutes

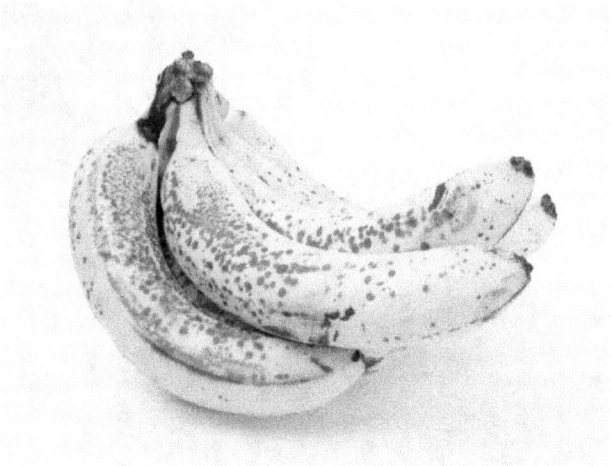

Ever wondered why bananas stay green in the tree and only starts to turn yellow after it has been picked?

It's because they are "climacteric," meaning the ripening is controlled by the banana's surrounding climate.

They show dramatic changes when they undergo the ripening (starch turns into sugar) process.

First, the green peel becomes yellow. Then as the banana reaches its ripe stage, brown flecks appear.

When the peel turns brown, then it is very ripe already.

I did not know anyone can hasten a banana's ripening until I became vegan.

Who could have thought that placing bananas in different corners of the house will make different results.

Turns out, the fastest way to ripen bananas is to put them in the oven.

Turn your oven at 250°F and let your banana sit there for 15 to 20 minutes. Once done, get your banana and observe what happened.

The low heat hastens the ripening, turning your starchy banana into a sweet one with mushy texture. However, this process turns the peel colour into black.

Extremely low temperatures work too. In just a few hours in the freezer, your banana will turn ripe and just like in the oven, the peel will turn black.

Now that you know how to ripe bananas in just a short time, you can now have your bananas in whatever stage of ripeness you'd like.

Want More?

Well, that was A LOT of information to swallow.

I hope you enjoyed reading it as much as I enjoyed writing it and are able to take some things with you.

The journey to veganism is definitely worthwhile but as I can attest to, is not always the easiest one.

To get products, recipes and other bonuses that have TRULY made my life easier, make sure to download the bonus pack which I'll continually update.

And if you enjoyed Vegan or Bust, would you mind taking a minute to leave a review on Amazon?

Even a short review helps and it'd mean a lot to me.

Until next time,

— Imran

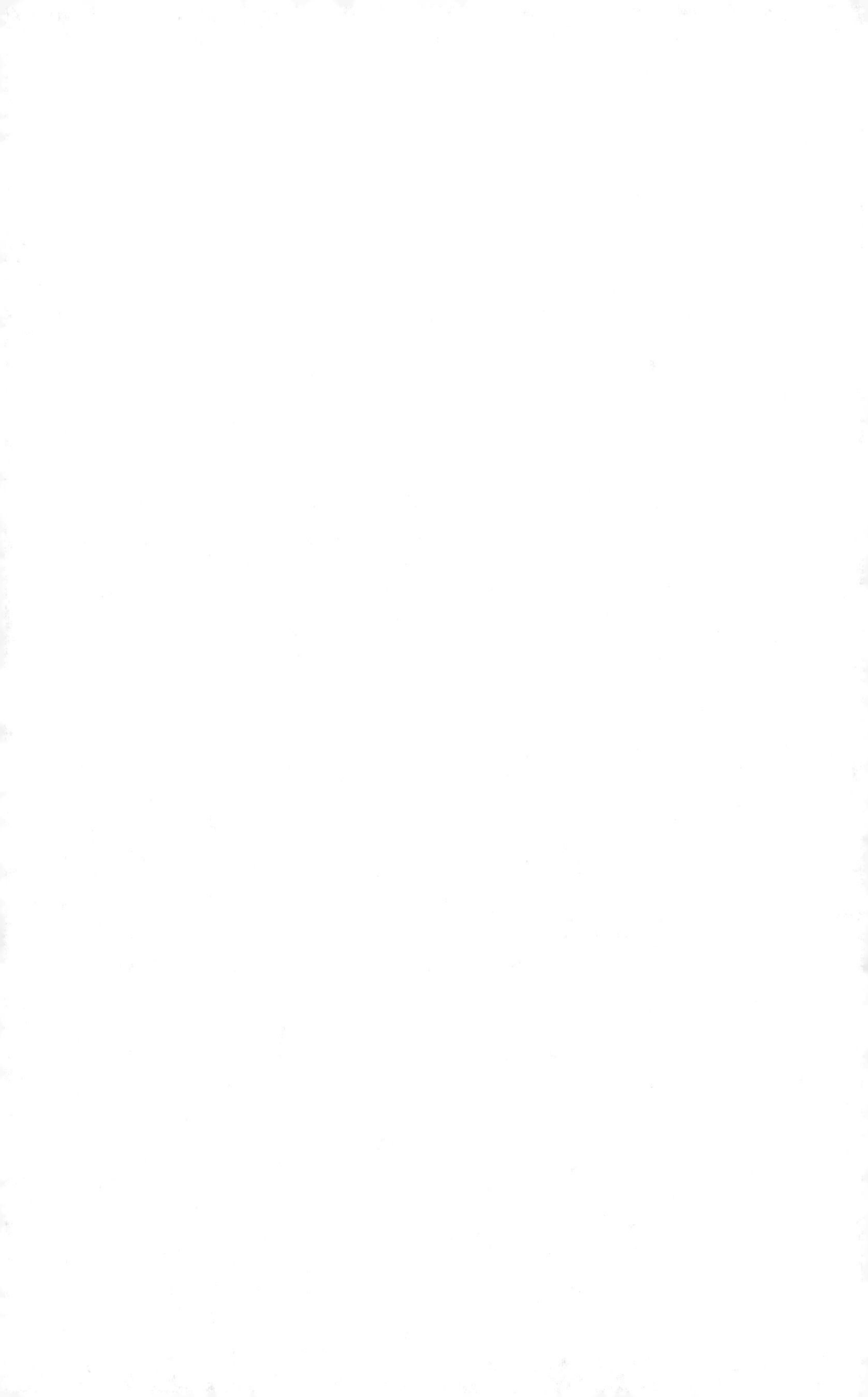